MASSAGEWORKS

MASSAGEWORKS

A Practical Encyclopedia of
Massage Techniques

by D. Baloti Lawrence
and Lewis Harrison

with Elinor Bowles

A GD/Perigee Book

Perigee Books
are published by
The Putnam Publishing Group
200 Madison Avenue
New York, NY 10016

Library of Congress Cataloging in Publication Data

Lawrence, D. Baloti.
   Massageworks: a practical encyclopedia of
massage techniques.

   "A GD/Perigee book."
   Bibliography: p.
   Includes index.
   I. Massage.   I. Harrison, Lewis.   II. Bowles,
Elinor.   III. Title.
RA780.5.L38   1983   615.8′22   82-21431
ISBN 0-399-50748-5

Illustrations by Fred Bush
Photographs by Ebet Roberts
Art consultation by Fred Spione

Designed by: ARLENE SCHLEIFER GOLDBERG

First Perigee printing, 1983
Printed in the United States of America
            7   8   9

To my mother, father, and family.

D. BALOTI LAWRENCE

To my mother, father, and the mystic guide and teacher who gave
me the vision to see all things as possible.

LEWIS HARRISON

Thanks Towan, Carolyn, Chaing, Sharnell, Michelle, Zanita, and Baloti for your love
and understanding; Paul Coates, Chuck Holden, Doria, Kenneth Moulden, Dr. Howard
Thurman, Leon Collins, Walter Hofer, Rehema Ellis, Kip Branch, Herman Clayborne,
D. Welling, Mr. and Mrs. L. L. Smith, and Dr. Doris Hall for your insight; and Lewis
Harrison, my most respected colleague, for sharing with me the next step.

D. BALOTI LAWRENCE

I would like to acknowledge the dear friends and associates who have contributed to
my development as a human being and teacher, including Vincent Collura, my first
teacher and the person who inspired my decision to enter this field; my sister Lilly
and her family; Dr. Randolph Stone, Alan Jay, Pierre Pannetier, and Dr. Sydney
Zerinsky, who all taught me the wonderful power of touch; Mark Becker and Leslie
Kaslof for their friendship and support over the years; Roberta Roll, who with her
clarity and patience was so important to my work; Phyllis Limpert and Robbie Fian;
and most important, D. Baloti Lawrence for sharing with me the next step.

LEWIS HARRISON

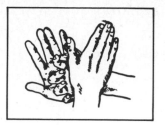

CONTENTS

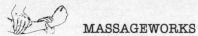 MASSAGEWORKS

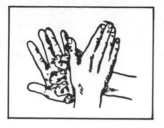

INTRODUCTION

If you awoke one morning with a muscle cramp, what would your first thought be? Get me an aspirin, a doctor, a tranquilizer? By the time you finish this book, you will understand that all of these answers are wrong.

Health care varies from country to country and from culture to culture, but through the ages massage has been part of nearly every medical system. Until early 1970s, massage was neglected in this country. Its greatest patrons were dancers, athletes, and members of health clubs and spas. Because of lack of knowledge about its wonderful therapeutic benefits the general public was deprived of the incredible benefits that massage can offer. But recently, the importance of hands-on healing arts have become universally recognized. Practitioners in every branch of the medical and healing professions believe that the recovery of patients may be quickened by massage.

As wonderful as the experience of a good massage may be, it should not be viewed as a sensual experience without therapeutic value. Hippocrates, considered the father of modern medicine, speaks highly of massage, especially in the treatment of difficulties of the joints. The ancient Greek writer Plutarch writes of the use of massage by Caesar. The indigenous peoples of Africa and North America employed massage, and in India there are specific massage techniques used on newborn babies. In the South Pacific the people of Tonga have specially trained massage practitioners, and it is considered among the highest of honors to receive a massage from one of them. Systematic massage came into use in the west during the

Renaissance. It had been popular for centuries in oriental and eastern countries, and by the late nineteenth and twentieth centuries massage techniques were commonly used by European doctors in the treatment of chronic diseases, especially those involving the nose and throat, certain heart ailments, and disturbances of the circulatory system.

Today, many health problems that were formerly treated with massage are instead placed under the care of physiotherapists. It is our belief, however, that there is a power and subtle healing quality from the skilled application of touch that cannot be equaled by any machine. The goal of this book is to offer you the opportunity to learn more about the healthgiving power of touch. But even more important than the power of touch is "being in touch" with your massage partner. Massage is much more than putting oil on someone's skin and then squeezing the muscles that seem tight. Sensitivity, warmth, and sharing are necessary ingredients to a good, therapeutic massage.

At the core of all high quality massage is rhythm. Just as a musician, gymnast, dancer, and assembly-line worker all need a profound sense of rhythm, a massage therapist's hands, breathing, and visualization must work together rhythmically.

When we first began to think about what we wanted to convey to our readers, we realized that there was no simple, concise massage book available that addressed the many health problems that can be solved with massage and that outlined a health maintenance program involving massage. As you turn these pages you will learn how to integrate a full health-building program using massage, exercise, water balancing, breathing, self-massage, and special energy balancing techniques. Now, on days when you feel sore and aching, you will have a guidebook to show you the fastest way to relief.

Action, knowledge, and love are the keys to life . . .

Action because it sparks our movement to get things done,

Knowledge because it expands the mind to show us what to do,

And love, because it embraces and warms the heart to bring happiness.

D. BALOTI LAWRENCE

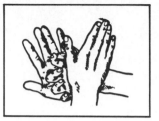

CHAPTER 1

MASSAGE AND BODYWORK SYSTEMS

When we feel pain, it's natural for us to rub the place that hurts. By rubbing our sore muscles or pressing our aching temples, we are trying, in our own instinctive way, to bring about a physical reaction that will correct the underlying disorder. We are, in effect, attempting body manipulation, more commonly known as massage.

The word "massage," which is derived from the Greek "masso" (I knead) and the Arabic "mass" (to press softly), is commonly used interchangeably with the body manipulation system known as Swedish massage. All too often this usage of the word massage confuses many "hands on" systems such as Rolfing, shiatsu, etc. with Swedish massage. We will use the terms "body manipulation," "bodywork," and "massage" interchangeably to refer to any of the hands on healing systems discussed in this book.

Many body manipulation systems exist, each having its own philosophy, techniques, health benefits, and limitations. The major philosophical distinction among body manipulation systems is whether they are structure-based or energy-based.

Structure-based systems, which arose for the most part from Western traditions of science and medicine, emphasize correcting the alignment of bones, muscles, and other connective tissue. These systems view the human body and its functioning in mechanical terms, merely as a "machine," without considering the subtle interactions between parts of the whole organism. Thus, these systems stress working with parts of the body that can be seen or functions that can be measured. Swedish massage, osteopathy, chiropractic, Rolfing, postural integration, and the Alexander Technique are examples of structure-based bodywork systems.

Energy-based systems start from the assumption that all living matter possesses a life-

1

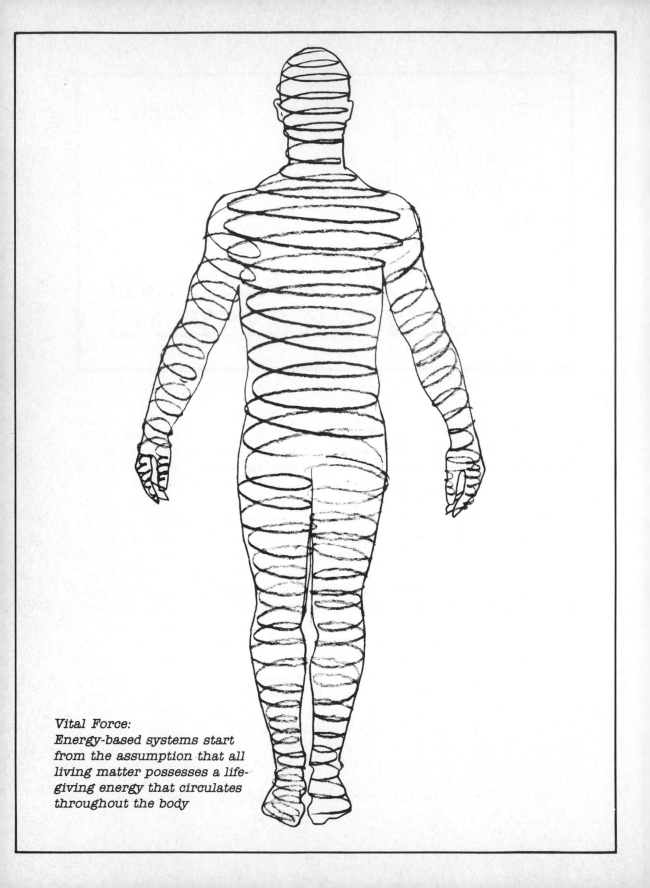

Vital Force:
Energy-based systems start
from the assumption that all
living matter possesses a life-
giving energy that circulates
throughout the body

giving energy or vital force that circulates throughout the body and must be kept strong and free-flowing to maintain health. In Japanese philosophy, this energy is called "ki"; in yoga it is called "prana." Names for this vital force in other systems include polarity, orgone, and magnetic fields. The mind and emotions, together with diet, exercise, and the air we breathe, influence the vitality of our energy system. When an imbalance or weakness in this vital force occurs, physical or emotional symptoms may result.

Energy-based systems are inspired essentially by Eastern philosophies of science and medicine that are more than 8,000 years old and can be traced back to Persia and the ancient Indian tradition of Ayurvedic medicine. Energy-based systems were also found among the healing philosophies of the Native Americans when Europeans first came to North America. These philosophies accept the existence of phenomena that can be experienced but cannot be seen or measured. Bodywork is only one of a number of tools that can be used to restore the body's energy balance. Acupressure, shiatsu, amma, and zone therapy are examples of energy-based systems.

Combined systems are a result of the convergence of Eastern and Western science. The meaning of vital force, or life energy, is becoming easier for Westerners to understand. It is known, for instance, that all matter, including our bodies, is composed of vibrating particles called atoms and that these particles give off light and heat energy that move in wavelike patterns. Consequently, there is a vibrational pattern to everything in nature. Albert Einstein provided a similar theoretical basis for the concept of vital force when he hypothesized that the entire universe is composed of mass energy, that there is a finite amount of this energy, and that it is constantly forming and reforming in new ways to create planets, stars, atmospheres, and living things. This concept of mass energy is similar to Eastern concepts of life energy or vital force. Through Western science we also know that our bodies are surrounded by magnetic fields. And Western medical practitioners now accept that the mind and emotions are important determinants of health. In addition, within the past decade, Western medicine has begun to accept the value of some Eastern healing systems such as acupuncture.

As a result of this relatively new integration of Eastern and Western medical and scientific concepts, several body manipulation systems have been created during the last eighty years that draw from both traditions. These systems recognize the importance of strengthening the life-energy system as well as correcting structural problems. Reichian therapy, bioenergetics, polarity, and our own system are examples of combined systems.

Bodywork systems—whether they are structure based, energy based or a combination of the two—use physical manipulation to stimulate the body's natural healing powers. With any of these systems, an individual can achieve the benefits of relaxation and pain relief. Moreover, body manipulation has fewer side effects, can be less expensive, and is more easily controlled than medication. This does not mean that massage should always be substituted for drugs or surgery, since there are many specific problems that are better approached by the latter two methods. Body manipulation is, however, a valuable medical tool that can in some instances be substituted for drugs and surgery and in other instances can be used as an adjunct to traditional medicine.

To get deep and lasting value from bodywork, however, you must strive to achieve a life style that is as healthy as possible. Unless you eat, rest, and exercise properly and maintain a positive mental attitude, massage will have only temporary, superficial effects.

The twenty-seven massage and bodywork systems presented in this chapter are loosely ordered from structural to energy based to combined and special systems. Popular techniques, such as Swedish massage, are discussed in greater depth than more esoteric techniques, such as Kahuna or Do-in.

Swedish Massage

Massage was at one time considered an essential part of Western medicine. In the fifth century B.C. Hippocrates wrote that every physician should learn body manipulation techniques. Galen, another physician of ancient Greece, wrote an entire book on the subject. The Romans used it in conjunction with bathing, probably as an early adjunct to hydrotherapy, which is the use of water to tone up or to sedate the muscles. Plutarch reported that Caesar received body manipulation regularly from a member of his staff.

Despite the early widespread popularity of massage, these techniques later fell into disrepute. Some writers on the subject believe this was because the early Church viewed the techniques as erotic rather than therapeutic. According to some historians, massagelike techniques went so far underground that they eventually could be found only in houses of prostitution.

This began to change in the last half of the sixteenth century with the writings of the French physician Ambroise Pare on the value of body manipulation to Western medicine. After him, other French surgeons and physicians began to explore body manipulation techniques and their benefits. Based on this knowledge, Henri Peter Ling, a student at the University of Stockholm, in Sweden, at the turn of the nineteenth century, created the system we know as Swedish massage.

Ling's purpose was to create a body manipulation system that would duplicate the movements of Swedish gymnastics and other types of exercise in order to stimulate circulation, increase muscle tone, and create an all-round balance to the structure and function of the muscle-skeletal system. Swedish gymnastics is an exercise regimen that includes bending, stretching, flexing, and rotating the muscles and joints to stimulate circulation. It contains 47 positions and over 800 movements. In Swedish massage, the practitioner imitates these exercise positions by using kneading, stroking, friction, tapping, and sometimes shaking or vibrating parts of the body. It can either stimulate or relax the body.

There are five classifications of manipulations in Swedish massage:

1. *Effleurage* (stroking). Long, centripetal strokes that may be deep or superficial. It heightens circulation, and acts to increase the blood flow to the area being massaged.

2. *Petrissage* (kneading). Picking up muscles, lifting them from the bones, and rolling, squeezing or wringing them. It is stimulating to the muscles and to circulation of the deeper blood vessels and lymphatics.

3. *Friction*. Circular rolling movement in treatment of joints and around bony prominences. It is useful in breaking down adhesions, promoting absorption of effusion, and in the relief of stasis. It raises local temperature, and should be followed by effleurage.

4. *Tapotement* (percussion). A technique performed in many ways such as hacking, clapping, tapping, beating and cupping. It is stimulating to the muscles and is either stimulating or calming to the nerves.

5. *Vibration*. A trembling movement of the tissues performed by the whole hand or the fingers. It has stimulating effect upon the nervous system by acting on the nerve centers or terminal nerve branches. Abdominal vibration is stimulating on the stomach, intestines and other digestive organs.

These techniques are most effective on the muscles, joints, nerves, and endocrine system. When used before an athletic workout, Swedish massage can prevent soreness, relieve swelling and tension, and improve muscular performance. By stimulating the circulation of blood and lymph, it can speed the body's rehabilitation from injury.

In spite of these benefits, Ling's new system was rejected by the Swedish government and the medical establishment. In 1812, when he applied for a license to teach and practice massage, he was told, "There are rope dancers and equestrian performers enough, without adding another one." Undaunted, Ling continued to practice massage, acquiring popular support and a number of influential clients who, it is believed, were instrumental in getting the government to reverse its decision and give him a license a year later, in 1813.

By the mid-1800s, the health effects of massage were recognized by many western physicians, and in Europe the masseur became a part of the health-care team, particularly in sports medicine. Americans were slower to recognize the validity of massage as a health-care technique, and by the end of the nineteenth century it was still not commonly used in this country. The general public was almost totally unaware of its benefits and there were few competent masseurs or schools to train them. The scarcity of the service made it expensive, and consequently it soon came to be regarded as a frivolous indulgence of the rich (an attitude that still persists to some degree).

The most important development for Swedish massage in this century has not been in techniques, which haven't changed much, but in the growing acceptance of massage as a therapeutic tool. Although there is a scarcity of recently published scientific studies on the clinical benefits of massage, most medical practitioners recognize its value. Today there are respected Swedish massage schools throughout the world, and many states in the United States have licensing procedures for practitioners of Swedish massage. And because there are many qualified practitioners, practically anyone can afford a massage.

Because it does not address an individual's nutritional, emotional, or biochemical state, which are essential components of health maintenance, Swedish massage is most effective when used in combination with other systems. As part of a total health program, Swedish massage can aid in bringing relief from stiffness, numbness, swelling, pain, constipation, and other health problems. Although some Swedish massage techniques can be done effectively on oneself and bring relief from tension and tired, aching muscles, most require a skilled practitioner.

Osteopathy

Osteopathy is a therapeutic system created by Dr. Andrew Taylor Still, an American physician who became disenchanted with traditional medicine after three of his sons died of spinal meningitis. In 1876, after sixteen years of study, Still presented his new system. The first college of osteopathy was founded in 1897. Although osteopathy began as an unorthodox system of medical treatment, it has become, in recent years, quite similar to conventional medical practice.

The underlying principle of osteopathy is that health problems result primarily from the derangement of the spinal column, which is composed of twenty-four movable vertebrae separated by pieces of cartilage called disks. These vertebrae shield the spinal cord. Dr. Still contended that when one or more of these vertebrae are displaced, they press on a nerve, resulting in the impairment of muscle and organ function and impeding or cutting off the flow of vital energy.

When a patient attempts to move a displaced vertebra, it locks, pressing on the associated disk. Over time the pressure can damage the disk, causing it to rupture. In conventional medicine, this condition is known as a herniated disk. Osteopaths call it an "osteopathic lesion." Herniated disks can be expected in those professions in which people sit in poor postures and develop weak stomach muscles. These can include truck, bus, or taxi drivers as well as people who sit in chairs all day. By manipulating the vertebra back into its proper position, the osteopath attempts to relieve the related nerve, muscle, and organ dysfunction.

Unlike chiropractors, osteopaths function virtually the same as medical doctors in office practice and in most states osteopaths are medical doctors under the licensing laws. Many of the athletes and dancers who would have gone to see osteopathic doctors in the early years of the twentieth century now go to physiotherapists, massage therapists, and chiropractors. Though it is not accurate to say that all osteopaths use medication in their treatments this trend had grown so wide by the 1960s that many patients who were wary of orthodox medical approaches became less inclined to see osteopaths. There is presently a new trend among osteopaths towards manipulation as a primary form of treatment though drug prescription is still widespread for health problems like headaches, backaches and other problems that respond well to body manipulation.

In osteopathy, body manipulation is a diagnostic as well as a treatment process. When trying to locate the osteopathic lesion that is the underlying cause of the patient's symptoms, the osteopath takes the limbs through a series of movements designed to restore the normal range of motion to impaired joints. When a previously locked joint opens, there is a clicking sound. It is believed by some osteopaths that this occurs because the pressure of the manipulation temporarily changes the lubricating fluid surrounding the joint from a liquid to a gaseous state, resulting in a temporary vacuum that makes a popping sound as it is being created.

Additional treatment depends on the extent and duration of the symptoms. The osteopath recognizes that for the relief afforded by manipulation to be truly lasting and effective, it must be supplemented with a balanced diet and other components of a health-building program. If the lesion is too serious to be relieved by manipulation and sound health habits alone, other treatments ranging from hydrotherapy to surgery may be recommended.

Cranial osteopathy, introduced by W.G. Sutherland, is one of the major sub-specialties created by osteopathic practitioners. Sutherland maintained that the skull is composed of tiny segments that can become locked into lesions that affect the brain and other parts of the body. Other osteopathic researchers have explored the effects of osteopathic treatment on the endocrine system.

Osteopathy has long been recognized as an effective method for relieving back and spinal problems, but it is also a system for treating all types of disease. Although treatment must be administered by a qualified practitioner, when it is part of a total health-care program, it can help you uncover your own natural healing powers.

Unlike some untraditional therapies, osteopathy has achieved almost the same acceptance from the public and the medical community as has orthodox medicine. Part of the reason for this acceptance is that over the years osteopathy has incorporated many aspects of traditional medicine, such as the use of drugs and surgery. And today, many osteopaths practice virtually without the use of manipulation. This is particularly true in the United States, where osteopaths function very much like other physicians. In countries such as England, however, traditional osteopathy is still widely practiced.

Osteopaths will treat virtually any health problem that an MD might treat. Osteopathic manipulation is highly suitable for athletic injuries and for injuries beyond the diagnostic skills of lay massage.

Chiropractic

Chiropractic was created by Daniel David Palmer, in 1895. Palmer based his system on principles outlined by the ancient Greek physicians and philosophers Hippocrates, Plato, Aristotle, Vesalius, and Galen, who traced health problems to the displacement of spinal vertebrae. The blockages in energy that occur when the vertebrae are misaligned are called "subluxations." Chiropractors attempt to relieve subluxations by adjusting the spine manually, as well as by counseling the patient on nutrition, exercise, and other components of a healthy life style. Some chiropractors claim that their approach allows patients more freedom than traditional medicine does in directing their own health care.

Chiropractic is recognized primarily as an effective therapy for back and spinal problems rather than as a total health-care system. Chiropractic is similar to osteopathy both in its focus on the condition of the spine and in its use of body manipulation for diagnosis and treatment of health problems. The two approaches are so similar that even some practitioners have trouble clearly explaining the differences between them because over the years osteopaths and chiropractors have found their various techniques often blend into one another's system. Many chiropractors practice osteopathic cranial manipulations and many osteopaths use the applied kinesiology system developed by Dr. George Goodheart, a chiropractor. One writer has said that, in fact, the only clear difference is that chiropractors are more likely to use X-rays as a diagnostic tool. Chiropractic, however, has not achieved the acceptance from the medical community that osteopathy has.

In spite of the continuing controversy surrounding chiropractic, some orthodox physicians have begun to explore the clinical value of the system. Most of the attention has been directed to its effectiveness in relieving musculoskeletal disorders. However, chiropractic has also been successful in bringing relief to patients with asthma, infertility, migraine headaches, and other nonskeletal problems.

Basically there are two types of chiropractors—those who do only spinal adjustments and those who view themselves as holistic health practitioners. The second group utilizes nutrition, hydrotherapy, iridology (iris diagnosis), colon irrigation, and other holistic techniques. This distinction, however, is not reflected in licensing requirements, which vary from state to state and determine what chiropractors are permitted to do.

Though chiropractors use varied techniques the general principle and application of the techniques is similar. It is seldom that a full chiropractic session will take place

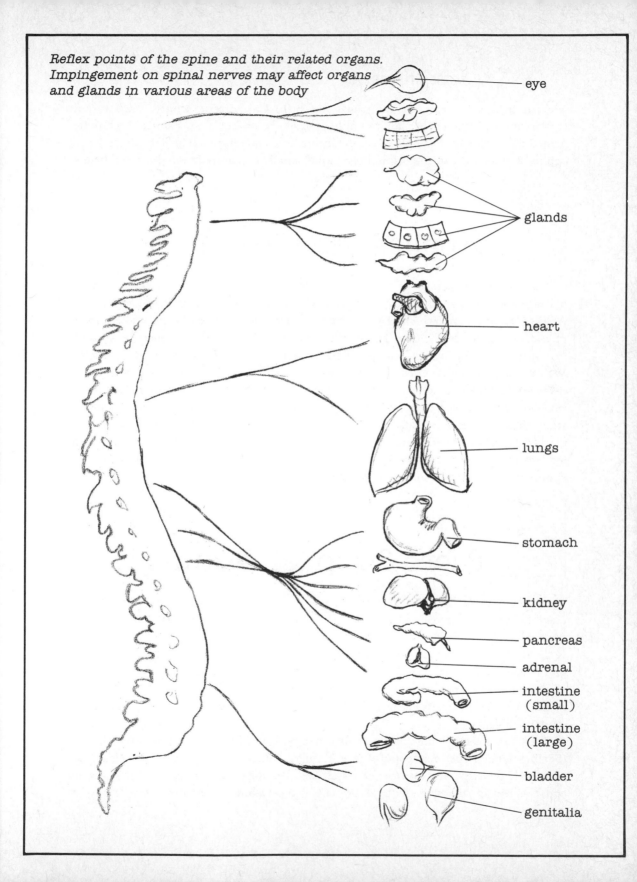

Reflex points of the spine and their related organs. Impingement on spinal nerves may affect organs and glands in various areas of the body

eye

glands

heart

lungs

stomach

kidney

pancreas

adrenal

intestine (small)

intestine (large)

bladder

genitalia

without some adjustment of the spinal vertebrae. Chiropractic schools teach various approaches to adjustment, for example, Logan Technique and Palmer Technique, named after schools of the same names. Included among chiropractic subspecialties are applied kinesiology, sacro-occipital technique, and TMJ manipulation described below.

Applied Kinesiology

Traditional kinesiology is the science of muscle anatomy and movement. When massage therapists speak of kinesiology, however, they are most probably speaking of Applied Kinesiology, which was developed by Dr. George Goodheart, a chiropractic physician, in the early 1960s. The system, known as A.K. to practitioners, is a highly systematic charting out of muscle reflexes and their effect on corresponding organs. When you go to an Applied Kinesiologist a series of "muscle tests" are performed to determine which muscles are strong or weak. The practitioner then recommends nutritional guidelines, prescribes herbs or applies acupressure or massage to various points to strengthen the weakened muscle or related organ. A more simplified version of A.K. is used by lay practitioners and some health professionals. This system is known as Touch for Health. Developed by John Thie, D.C., from Dr. Goodheart's work, it is an easily applied and practical system of self-health care.

Sacro-Occipital Technique

Orthodox medicine has paid little attention to the role that the position of the eight cranial bones plays in maintaining good health and physical and emotional balance. The bone which seems to have one of the greatest effects on the position of the cranial bones is the mandible (lower jaw bone). In every facial movement, the mandible moves much of the face and skull. When the lower jaw bone is misaligned, this will affect the alignment of the other cranial bones. This chain reaction can result in many major and minor health problems from lower back pain, headaches, and facial neuralgia to various dental problems.

There are several techniques for cranial manipulation, but Sacro-Occipital Technique (SOT) is among the most popular. The technique is practiced primarily by chiropractors, orthodontists, and osteopathic physicians. Developed primarily through the work and theories of Major B. DeJarnette, D.C., the technique enables properly trained practitioners to perform cranial examinations and determine and correct cranial bone imbalances. SOT also involves techniques for the sacral and occipital bones as they affect cranial bone balance.

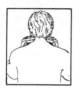

Temporomandibylar Joint Technique (TMJ)

In the early part of this century, dentists began to notice that many symptoms, including pains in the neck, ears and head, dizziness, and ringing in the ears, could be tied to structural problems in the temporomandibular joint (the joint that forms the jaw). TMJ technique has different schools of thought and treatment approaches, many of them overlapping. Chiropractors, dentists, osteopaths and orthopedists have different opinions about the causes of TMJ imbalance and the most effective approach to the problem. Emotional stress, dental malocclusion (a jaw shift initiated by misaligned teeth which causes muscle spasms in the jaw), osteoarthritis, as well as nutritional factors in childhood are all thought to cause structural problems leading to TMJ imbalance. No one TMJ technique has been shown to be "universal" in correcting these imbalances. TMJ techniques are all effective depending on the case and specific client needs (see page 120).

Alexander Technique

In the 1880s a young Australian actor named Frederick Matthias Alexander inexplicably lost his voice one night on stage. After consulting with a number of physicians, and after none of the medications and other treatments they prescribed worked, he retired from the theater and spent the following ten years examining the way he used his body when speaking and acting. He noticed that when he opened his mouth to speak, he involuntarily pulled his head back and down. This was part of a pattern that included lifting his chest, hollowing his back, and making dozens of other small involuntary movements. For ten years he worked in front of a mirror to correct each of these movements.

From this experience he created the Alexander technique of body awareness to help others learn more efficient and less destructive ways of using their bodies. A crucial movement in the Alexander technique is learning to lift the head and neck properly. This results in an improvement in "posture," an expansion of the chest cavity, and allowing the internal organs room to function. It can aid in bringing relief from high blood pressure, joint and muscle pain, as well as the loss of the voice.

Many prominent people, including John Dewey, a leading educational theorist, and playwright George Bernard Shaw, have studied the Alexander technique and testified to its benefits. Both men lived past the age of ninety and gave the Alexander technique at least part of the credit for their longevity. Alexander himself continued to teach his system until his death in 1955, at the age of eighty-six.

The Alexander technique is used by many dancers and actors, since proper use of voice and movement results from regular practice of Alexander movements. Alexander techniques also can improve breathing and increase body movement efficiency. An Alexander teacher might diagnose a golfer's failure to produce a good stroke, for example, as due to misdirection of general body mechanics.

The Alexander technique is taught and practiced at schools throughout the world. It is an excellent self-awareness system that, in order to produce the maximum benefit, should be part of a total health program.

A person must be patient with Alexander technique for the sessions can occasionally be slow moving. The sessions involve repeated guided body movement as well as table work massage techniques. However, this constant repeating of specific body movements is necessary to achieve the desired goal of greater freedom of movement and postural balance and should not be viewed as a negative aspect of the system. Many people who have experienced voice problems as well as foot, back, and general postural imbalances have received great benefit from the Alexander technique.

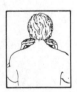

Mensendieck

This system was developed by Dr. Elizabeth Mensendieck, an American who had studied medicine in Switzerland. She began working with medical problems associated with impaired muscle function. Initially, her work involved a series of experiments with paralyzed and semi-paralyzed patients whom she helped regain muscular activity and control by visualization and will power exercises. About 1905, she developed an exercise system which bears her name. The system is much more well-known in Europe than in the U.S. However, in the 1930s, the championship swimming team at Yale was given Mensendieck exercise training. Lessons are usually a half-hour, are done in the nude (men wear jock straps) and all sessions are done one-on-one. There are a number of areas where Alexander and Mensendieck approaches may seem similar, but the techniques are essentially different. This system has gained great respect for the success it has in curing various painful structural problems.

Rolfing

Many of us can remember being admonished as children to "stand up straight." The general rule was "shoulders back, stomach in, head up." Actually, according to Ida Rolf, PhD, the creator of the Rolf System of Structural Integration, this posture misaligns the spine and deforms the skeleton.

In Dr. Rolf's system, gravity is the "great healer." When the skeleton is not vertical, the body expends energy resisting the pull of gravity. In Rolfing, manipulation is used to realign the skeleton and make it vertical, which, according to Rolfers, makes the individual feel lighter and more graceful. When the body's structure is corrected, basic chemical changes take place within the body that improve overall health.

The Rolfer's ability to realign the skeleton stems from the fact that the body is a "plastic medium"—a collection of segments (head, thorax, pelvis, legs) and not a single unit, as traditionally viewed by Western medicine. Rolfing straightens the body by correcting relationships between the segments. The Rolfer accomplishes this by performing deep manipulation of the connective tissue, collagen. As do other proteins, collagen changes from a solid to a gel-like substance when heat or mechanical energy is applied. When the Rolfer manipulates the skeleton, the hands generate energy that loosens the collagen and makes it more pliable.

Rolfers believe that distortions in the skeleton can have a number of causes, including physical and emotional trauma. A person who has suffered such trauma may hold the body in a defensive, rigid position. When that person is Rolfed, the initial trauma may surface, releasing blocked emotional energy. A good Rolfer should be trained to handle the deep emotional experiences that can be unleashed.

Rolfing is an excellent technique for correcting skeletal misalignment, but Rolfing can be used to treat anything from releasing long-term emotional trauma to realigning major posture problems such as scoliosis (lateral curvature of the spine). Many problems not directly viewed as musculoskeletal by physicians may appear to be temporarily or permanently relieved after Rolfing. Whether this is due to a release of emotional trauma or an unknown factor cannot be easily determined.

Rolfing sessions can be somewhat more costly than other bodywork techniques (from $50 to $100 per session). A Rolfing treatment involves ten sessions.

The Rolfing process can also be very physically painful, depending on the Rolfer's individual sensitivity to the client and the amount of client resistance.

In all fairness, most people we have spoken to have considered their Rolfing experience to be a positive one in spite of the pain and discomfort experienced during the sessions.

Amma

Eastern body manipulation techniques started in India and made their way into China and had spread to Korea and Japan by the eighth century A.D. They are based on the theory that there are vital points, *tsubo,* on the body, which are connected by meridians, or *keraku,* that are channels of life energy between the skin and internal organs. The *amma* practitioner presses these vital points (tsubo) with the fingers, elbows, knuckles, and feet.

Until the seventeenth century *amma* was widely used throughout Asia. It gradually lost credence, however, because many people began to regard it more as a pleasure than a therapy, a view that persisted until the nineteenth century. During that period, techniques based on *amma,* such as *shiatsu* and *kahuna,* were developed. Today, however, *amma* is one of the three manipulation systems practiced in Japan. (*Shiatsu* and Swedish massage are the other two.)

A basic principle of *amma* is that muscles and skin become tense as a result of congestion in the circulatory system, caused by stagnant blood. Just as Swedish massage does, amma releases that stagnation by stimulating the heart rate and blood flow. Practitioners stress motions away from the heart toward the limbs.

Amma, which can be performed by someone else or as a self-care technique, is deeply relaxing, and is effective in bringing relief from fatigue, sluggishness, swelling, stiff shoulders, chilling in the hands and feet, and headaches. Best results are obtained when it is used as part of a total health program.

However, you will find fewer practitioners of *amma* in the United States than of its more common relatives, *shiatsu* or Swedish massage.

Shiatsu and Acupressure

Shiatsu, a word meaning finger *(shi)* and pressure *(atsu),* is a Japanese bodywork system derived from amma and the Chinese system Do-In. As with other energy-based systems, shiatsu and acupressure are used to improve the flow of *ki,* or energy, in the body. Along with food, air, water, and exercise, shiatsu and acupressure release the *ki*, which emanates from the body's main energy center, which is located one inch below the navel, and travels throughout the body along defined pathways.

Both *shiatsu* and acupressure involve the pressing of vital points and energy meridians firmly with the fingers, thumbs, and palms to diagnose and bring relief from health problems. Many of these points are the same as those identified by acupuncturists. Acupressure differs from *shiatsu* in that it consists mainly of pressure-point therapy. In *shiatsu,* the practitioner also manipulates various parts of the body.

An important difference between *shiatsu* and acupressure and many other bodywork systems is the philosophy of *yin* and *yang,* which is at the core of the concept of *ki*. In oriental philosophy, the universe represents the interplay of opposing forces that attract each other and must be kept in dynamic balance: negative and positive electrical energy; work and rest; male and female energy; the inward pull of gravity and the outward spread of the solar system.

Yang forces are classified as hot, active, energetic, outreaching and male. Yin forces are classified as cold, dark, slow-moving, inward-looking, and female. Yin and yang are always relative. For example, New York in the winter may be yin (cold) in comparison

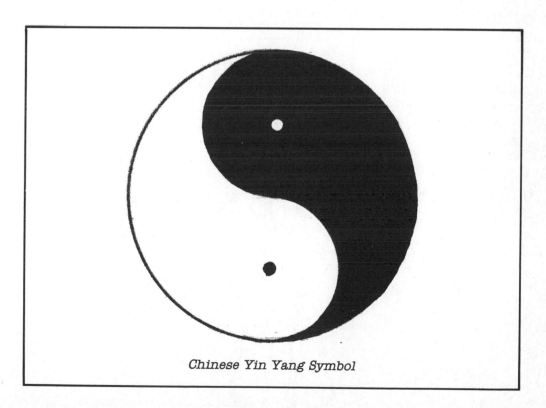

Chinese Yin Yang Symbol

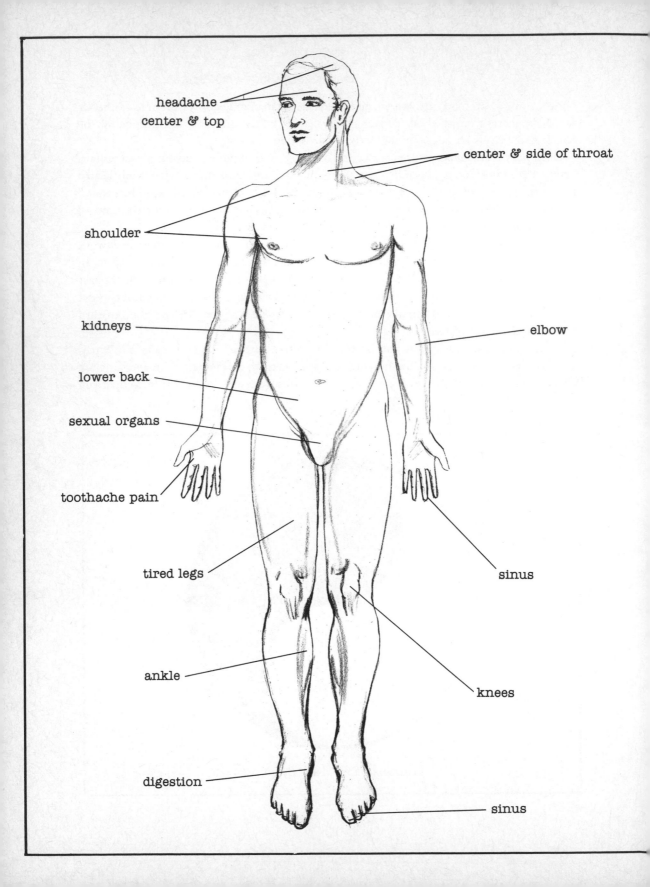

headache
center & top

center & side of throat

shoulder

kidneys

elbow

lower back

sexual organs

toothache pain

tired legs

sinus

ankle

knees

digestion

sinus

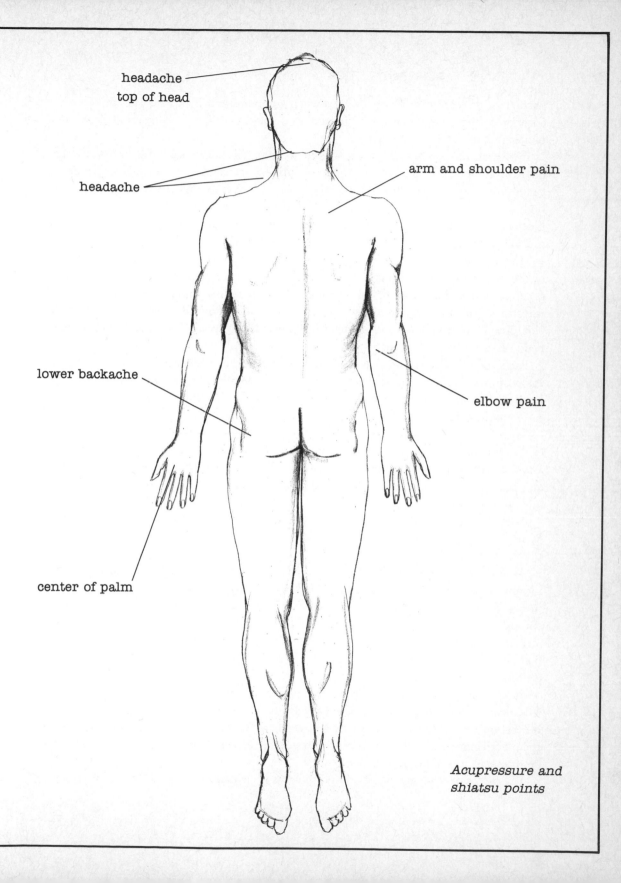

headache
top of head

headache

arm and shoulder pain

lower backache

elbow pain

center of palm

*Acupressure and
shiatsu points*

with California, but it is yang (warm) when compared with Alaska. The universe is a constantly changing mixture of yin and yang, and the key to balancing them is to maintain their proper proportions.

In shiatsu and acupressure, the goal is to maintain the balance and proper distribution of *ki* throughout the body. When there is an illness or disorder, some organs, glands, or tissues may have too much *ki,* while others may not have enough. By manipulating the body's vital points and meridians, the shiatsu or acupressure practitioner can clear blockages that may be impeding the proper flow of ki. Blockages may be indicated by muscle tightness, pain in movement or limited range of movement.

Understanding the movement of *ki,* which varies according to the form and structure of the body's organs, is essential to shiatsu or acupressure evaluation and therapy. Each organ is classified as either hollow or solid. From the hollow organs (the large and small intestines, gall-bladder, stomach, and bladder), the *ki* flows downward toward earth. The flow of *ki* from the solid organs (the lungs, liver, spleen, pancreas, kidneys, and heart) is toward the heavens.

Each organ is also classified as an element, according to the density of its vital energy. According to Taoist philosophers, there are five elements in all creation: wood, fire, earth, water, and metal. Each of these elements has a different vital-energy level and a different function.

The movement of one element to the next is a cycle of generation, known as the *sheng* cycle, which is shaped like a circle. Wood burns in fire. Fire creates earth by making ashes. Earth, over time, turns into metal ore. But metal is composed of air and mud, and mud is made up of earth and water. Water in turn gives life to plants and trees, which create wood.

There is also a parallel cycle of the flow of energy, known as *ki,* which is star shaped. Water puts out fire, fire melts metal, metal cuts wood, and wood, in the form of the plow, conquers the soil.

According to the *shiatsu*/acupressure classification system, the heart is a fire organ, the kidney is a water organ, the liver is a wood organ, the spleen is an earth organ, and the lungs are metal. If a patient's heart center is overworked, the practitioner can sedate it through the *ki* cycle by manipulating points related to the kidney, which is a water element capable of dousing the heart's fire. Conversely, if the lung meridian, which is metal, lacks *ki,* the practitioner may follow the *sheng* cycle and manipulate the spleen center, which is earth.

Each organ also has a daily cycle of activity that influences the therapeutic process. The heart center, for example, is relatively inactive when we wake up. The bladder center, on the other hand, is usually full when we wake up. In shiatsu and acupressure the practitioner does not place as much pressure on an active organ, such as a full bladder or stomach, as on an inactive organ.

The direction and flow of *ki,* or vital force, is of primary importance when the shiatsu or acupressure practitioner is working on a specific health problem. But other factors that can have a bearing on an individual's health—personal habits, emotional or personality traits, height, weight, and other physical measurements, and occupation—must also be taken into account in evaluation and therapy.

Recently scientists have discovered that the body produces natural painkillers called endorphins. Energy-based systems like *shiatsu,* acupressure, and polarity (see page 1) can stimulate the release of these chemicals through the nervous system. Two parts of the nervous system—the sympathetic and the parasympathetic—work together to regulate other body systems and organs. The sympathetic nervous system excites the body and alerts it to impending danger. The parasympathetic system calms the body when the danger has passed. *Shiatsu* can act either on the sympathetic nervous system to increase circulation (tone up) or on the parasympathetic nervous system to lower blood pressure (sedate). (See page 54 for more information about the nervous system.)

For the *shiatsu* practitioner, there is no difference between diagnosing a problem and prescribing a therapy. For example, if a particular part of the body has too much vital energy, the therapy is to sedate it. The four major evaluation or diagnostic tools in shiatsu are observation, listening, questioning, and touch.

Observation (bo shin) involves looking at the eyes, hands, fingernails, tongue, and face-reading. In face-reading each part of the face reveals something about the condition and history of a part of the body. A person with horizontal lines across the forehead, for example, is lacking in energy. Vertical lines across the forehead indicate overeating. Large circles under the eyes may denote a kidney imbalance or that the patient drinks too many liquids. Excessive facial hair, especially on a woman, may be the result of consuming too many dairy products. The lower lip reflects the condition of the intestines; the upper lip reflects the stomach. Even the shape of the face and the size of the nostrils provide information about the condition of internal organs.

Listening (bun-shin) to the heart and other organs of the body is the second major evaluation tool. It also means listening to the patient's tone of voice and being sensitive to his or her mood.

When questioning a patient *(mon-shin),* the practitioner asks for an assessment of what might be wrong and for information about the patient's life style, working conditions, and other individual characteristics.

The fourth tool, touch *(setu-shin),* is a crucial technique in shiatsu. One *setu-shin* evaluation method, pulse reading, involves touching the main energy center in the body—the source of all *ki.* (In Japan there are shiatsu specialists who work only with this energy center.)

In Asia *shiatsu* techniques have been a part of popular self-care systems for thousands of years. In Japan *shiatsu* practitioners, along with Swedish massage and amma practitioners, are licensed. In the United States during the last ten years, *shiatsu* has become popular both as a self-care system and as a service rendered by professional practitioners.

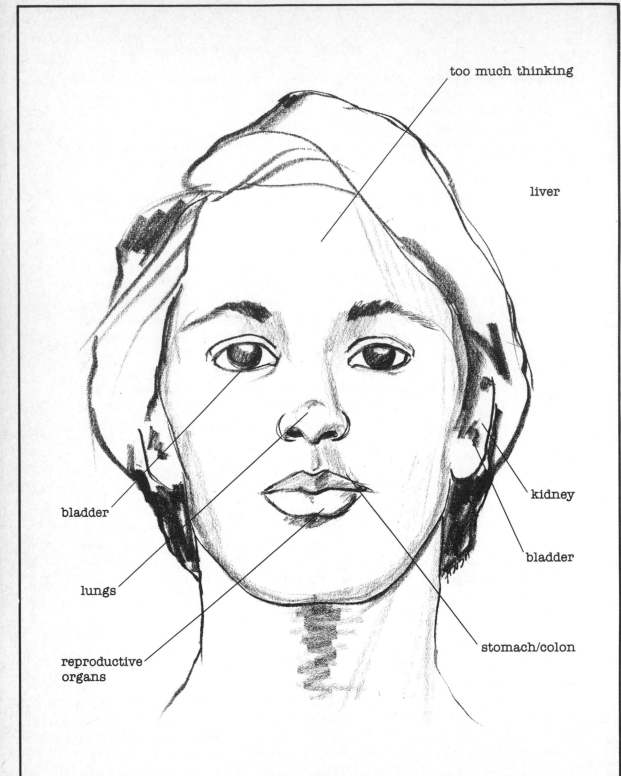

too much thinking

liver

bladder

kidney

lungs

bladder

reproductive
organs

stomach/colon

Face-reading diagnosis chart

When stress, hypertension, headaches, or insomnia is a problem, *shiatsu* is a powerful technique. It is especially useful because individuals can apply the various techniques to themselves on a daily basis.

Do-In

Do-In is a highly respected self-massage technique which traces its origins from Japan. The most important techniques used in the system are similar to those that are applied in Shiatsu (see page 14). Many Do-In points are located on the feet, neck, face and cranium. The Do-In system is especially useful for emotional stress, mental fatigue and tension headaches.

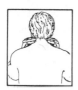

Kahuna

Kahuna is an energy-based healing system that originated in Hawaii and the Philippines. Some Kahuna practitioners hardly touch the body, and, in a sense, are practicing a "laying on of hands." The Philippine Kahuna practitioners may do a session using the balls of their feet instead of their hands. Generally, the recipient of a Kahuna session will have an experience of increased energy flow and vitality throughout the body as well as a relaxed state of mind. In comparing Kahuna work to other systems, it is probably closest to Shiatsu or Amma therapy.

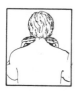

Chua K'a ©*

Chua K'a advocates point out that we are born soft and flexible, and that as we age our bodies acquire debilitating tensions. *Chua K'a,* which means "to sculpture out," is an ancient Mongolian body manipulation system based on the theory that the muscles "remember" earlier traumas and painful experiences. The traumas, and the muscular tensions they produce, will remain until they are released from the body.

---

*Chua K'a is a service mark of Arica Institute, Inc. © 1973 Arica Institute, Inc.

The system is said to have come from techniques used by Genghis Khan's warriors. The pain and fear they had stored from battle wounds lingered until released through body manipulation. *Chua K'a* was developed in its present form and was introduced to the United States by Oscar Ichazo, a teacher of the Arica System of Human Development. *Chua K'a* is not for people who are under extreme emotional imbalance, but it is greatly appreciated by people who wish to clean out the nooks and crannies of past tension. *Chua k'a* is especially useful for those who have old physical injuries.

The treatment begins with the "rolling" of the skin in long, vertical strokes. This helps to remove cellulite, which is stored in fatty globules under the skin. It also helps increase circulation and return elasticity to the skin, resulting in a more youthful appearance. The second step involves deep manipulation of muscles and bones. By relaxing muscles at the points at which the tendons attach them to the bone, *Chua K'a* enables the body to operate more freely, with the muscles and bones working against each other. In *Chua K'a,* the body is said to have twenty-seven regions. Each region stores a different psychological fear. For example, the lower back stores fear of losing; the upper back and shoulders contain fears of being burdened; the scalp collects worries and preoccupations; the thighs become lumpy when we feel inadequate. As the *Chua K'a* treatment proceeds, the body relaxes and often releases the initial trauma, thereby clearing the way for positive emotions. Women with cellulite and people who experience great fear and aches and pains that are associated with emotional stress will find this the technique of choice.

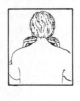

Zone Therapy and Reflexology

At the beginning of this century, an American physician, Dr. Edwin F. Bowers, and his contemporaries George Starr White, MD, and William H. Fitzgerald, MD, identified a system of zones throughout the body. These zones consist of points that affect the vital energy traveling to various body parts. They end in the feet, and their end points can be manipulated to balance blocked energy pathways in the body. Although there are zones in the ears and other parts of the body, the primary focus of zone therapy and reflexology has been on the hands and feet. Reflexology and zone therapy are very similar in application, however, practitioners of reflexology are found throughout the United States while zone therapy practitioners are few and far between. This is probably because of the increasing popularity of shiatsu, polarity therapy, and acupressure which have a

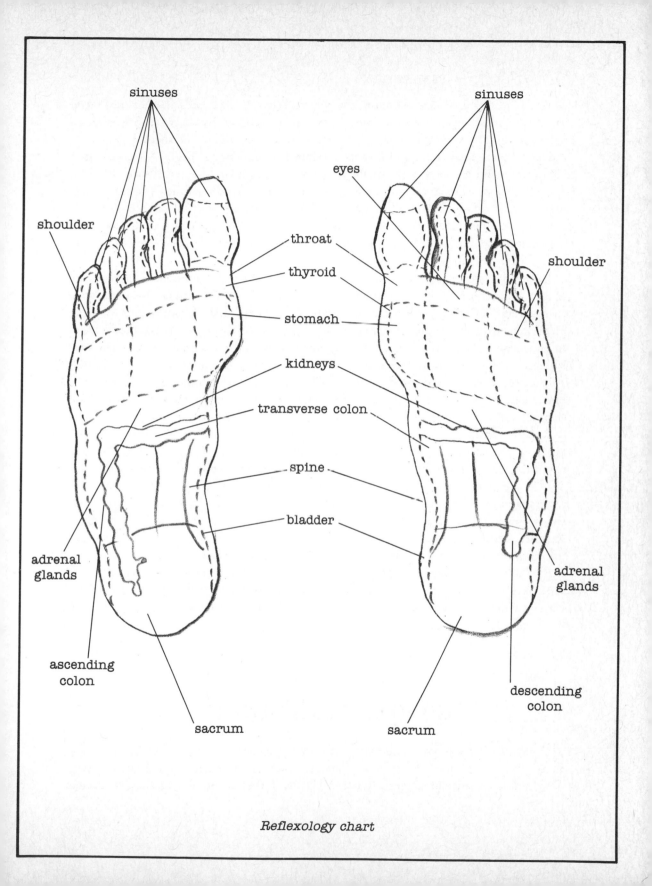

Reflexology chart

much more sophisticated reasoning for the structure of the zones in their respective systems. Reflexology also focuses much more on the relationship between points found on the soles of the feet and reflexes throughout the body than zone therapy does.

Drs. White, Fitzgerald, and Bowers developed the following theory: When a person applies pressure to the feet, he or she may notice a granular texture beneath the skin. Areas with extensive granulation are the most sensitive to the applied pressure. They believed that this granular texture was a result of uric-acid crystallization in the feet. By rubbing the crystals on the nerve endings in the soles, a reaction is initiated between these zones and associated organs and glands throughout the body. These reactions were called reflex reactions.

Eastern physicians consider diagnosis through the feet to be an essential prerequisite to the proper use of herbs, acupuncture, and associated therapies. However, zone therapy and reflexology were dismissed when they were first introduced to Western physicians, probably because the conceptual origins of the theory were difficult for them to understand. This attitude has changed somewhat with the acceptance of acupuncture. Interestingly, however, neither acupressure nor reflexology has gained the following that acupuncture has achieved in recent years. While acupuncture is almost always done by a practitioner, people can easily use reflexology and other finger-pressure methods on themselves.

Reflexology is one of a number of therapeutic systems whose physical basis is only beginning to be understood. Many orthodox physicians in the United States still question the value of foot reflexology because they have not been able to verify whether the crystals are in fact uric acid in origin. Whatever the chemical composition may be of these granules, which can easily be felt by rubbing your thumb on the soles of your feet, they do exist. And thousands of experiences have shown that there is a direct relationship between the breakdown of these crystals and the relief of arthritic pain, constipation, back pain, and many other health problems. Since the feet serve as reflexes for the entire body, reflexology is an appropriate technique in all situations. However, it is best used in conjunction with other massage systems. Reflexology is especially good for those who experience general aches and pains, and the technique is especially useful in bringing relief to headaches and sinus congestion.

 # Therapeutic Touch

Touch is a very common and meaningful way of sharing our feelings with others, and in the healing professions, such as nursing, touch is an invaluable therapeutic tool. Carvings from ancient Egypt, India, Tibet, and the medieval churches of Roman

Catholicism illustrate that the "laying on of hands" has been valued for centuries.

The underlying premise of therapeutic touch is that health is promoted when the exchange of energy between an individual and his or her environment is balanced. This energy, called *prana* in Sanskrit, is the same as *ki* or vital force. The word *prana* is derived from *pra* (forth) and *na* (to breathe, to move, or to live). By passing his or her hands lightly over the patient's body, the healer can feel any energy imbalances, which usually show up as one of several sensations: heat, cold, tingling, pulsation, electric shock, or tightness. When an imbalance is felt, the healer can redirect the energy by will.

Until very recently, because the physical basis of therapeutic touch has been difficult to test or understand scientifically, its value has been largely discounted by the medical profession. There has, however, been some research that demonstrates the value of this method. In 1964 Bernard Grad, a biochemist at McGill University, in Canada, did a series of experiments with healer Oskar Estabany. Grad soaked barley seeds in a salty solution to make them "sick," and then divided them into experimental and control groups. He had Estabany hold some flasks of water in the same way he did when laying on hands, and used this water on seeds in the experimental group. He poured regular water on the control group. Grad found that the seeds in the experimental group grew faster, produced sprouts with a greater net weight, and held more chlorophyll than did those in the control group.

In 1971, after reviewing Grad's research, Dolores Krieger, RN, PhD, conducted the first of three pilot studies on the biochemical effect of therapeutic touch on humans. She used an experimental group of patients who received touch healing and a control group that did not. Again, Oskar Estabany was the healer. She monitored the patients' hemoglobin. In each of these pilot tests, the experimental group's hemoglobin count rose dramatically, while in the untreated group, the hemoglobin counts remained largely unchanged. Krieger concluded that a transfer of energy had taken place between Estabany and his patients, and that because hemoglobin is sensitive to oxygen, it reflected the energy transfer. Her hypothesis is based on the concept of *prana,* which refers to the life breath emanating from the sun and sent out from the spiritual plane to all other levels of existence.

Krieger continued her studies with larger groups of patients in 1972, 1973, and 1974, the last with the support of the American Nurses' Association Council of Nurse Researchers. In the last study, nurses acted as healers. Each of the studies confirmed her earlier results.

Since 1975, Krieger has been teaching classes in therapeutic touch at New York University Nursing School, where she obtained her own training. Therapeutic touch is now part of the curriculum at more than thirty nursing schools around the country.

Proskauer Massage

Developed by Magda Proskauer, this massage system uses a very light touch, and places great emphasis on the client's breathing rhythm in relation to the massage process. Although it is not in wide use, this system is powerful because of the internal massage effect created by the breathing rhythm. It is, in a sense, both inner and outer massage.

Reichian Therapy

Wilhelm Reich (1898–1957), an Austrian psychoanalyst, combined bodywork with Freudian psychoanalysis. He used manipulation to dissolve the structural disorders in the body that he called "body armor" and which he considered to be physical manifestations of blocked emotional energy.

Like Freud, with whom he worked from 1922 to 1928 as a clinical assistant at the Vienna Psychoanalytic Polyclinic, Reich believed that emotional, mental, and physical disorders are caused by sexual repression. He argued that because Western society condemned the basic sexual urges that are an integral part of the human experience, we fight our sexual feelings. The blocked sexual energy, which affects our other emotions as well, expresses itself in destructive and neurotic behavior in situations in which we feel vulnerable or threatened by the loss of control. The goal of Reichian therapy is to have the patient release these repressed sexual and emotional energies. Once this release occurs, according to Reich, the individual is free to experience and accept the full range of his or her sexuality and emotions, and live a freer, healthier life.

Reichian therapy has seven major components designed to dissolve body armor. The therapeutic process progresses from the superficial to the deepest defenses of the individual.

The first component is deep breathing and repeated screaming, which can sometimes produce emotional release by itself. This release takes place in convulsive, orgasmlike waves. The second component is deep tissue manipulation, which is done while the patient acts out his or her physical or emotional pain with the face, voice, or body. The purpose of this is to trigger the memory and release of earlier emotional traumas.

Third, the therapist has the client make unusual faces and sounds. Often a set facial expression will be a part of the individual's body armor. For example, someone who smiles when relating tragic events is probably blocking his or her true feelings. Fourth, an analyst pushes on the patient's chest while the client screams.

Fifth, the analyst pays close attention to the patient's cough, gag, and yawning reflexes. These are considered "release responses" that indicate the unblocking of pent-up emotions. Sixth, the analyst forces the patient to stay in stressful positions in order to help the patient become uncomfortable with his or her own armoring.

Finally the therapist encourages "bioenergetic movements"—kicking, stamping, tantrums—to release pent-up anger and energy.

Reich hypothesized that the major energy blocks are located in seven segments throughout the body: around the eyes, the mouth, the neck, the chest (including the arms), the diaphragm, the abdomen, and the pelvis (including the legs). These segments are independent, but decreased armoring in one segment may result in increased armoring in another, as a way of compensating. (The idea of compensation occurs in other energy-based systems. In shiatsu, for example, if one energy center contains too much *ki,* some other energy center usually has too little.)

Reichian bodywork produces emotional releases that are then reinforced with other aspects of the therapy. As the therapy progresses, the patient is expected to carry out its principles in his or her life.

Although the value of the Reichian system is now largely unquestioned, Reich's views originally were resisted by members of the medical establishment. However, many people who accept the concept of energy-based systems disagree with his underlying hypothesis that all blocked emotion is sexual in nature. Reich died in 1957 in a penitentiary, after his long-running conflicts with orthodox medicine led to his prosecution and conviction on charges of fraudulent medical practices. Reich's work and theories are generally held in high regard by most bodywork practitioners, and he is considered by many to simply have been a man ahead of his time.

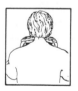

Feldenkrais

The bodywork system developed by Moshe Feldenkrais, Israeli physicist and associate of Joliot-Curie, addresses the interaction of emotional and physical patterns. Each of us speaks, moves and thinks in a different way, according to the self image we develop over the years. Each action we perform is composed of four major components—movement, sensation, feeling, and thought. Optimal functioning requires a balance of all four. As we leave childhood, our actions tend to be more and more governed by societal pressures, organization, and "accepted" images. These factors limit the development of our full potential and foster the growth of set patterns of thought, action and feeling.

In order to change the way we act, we must change our self image and the motivations tied to it. Dr. Feldenkrais believes that awareness of our actions is the key to overcoming habitual patterns of thought and action and expanding our capabilities. Movement is the ideal medium in which to effect changes and is directly tied to the nervous system and all our actions, thoughts, and feelings.

Through simple body manipulation and exercises, changes are achieved in the motor cortex, which effect changes in muscular patterns and the thought and feeling patterns associated with them. By learning to feel and sense what is going on, we can discover changes within ourselves. By integrating breathing with movement and by concentrating on improving our ability and going beyond our self-imposed boundaries, we can eliminate superfluous actions and realize our full potential.

Polarity

Polarity draws on Western and Eastern theories that assume the existence of energy fields in the body that must be balanced to maintain health. These fields may be called bioenergy, *ki,* orgone, or vital force. Health is a delicate balance of physical, mental, and emotional energy. When disease occurs, there is a blockage or disruption in the flow of energy through the body.

Dr. Randolph Stone, the creator of the polarity system, began in the early 1900s to study chiropractic, osteopathy, naturopathy, acupuncture, reflexology, and other health systems from around the world. Dr. Stone concluded that the human body is more than muscles, glands, and nerves. He believed that a magnetic field directed these grosser systems. He took these different healing programs, which included herbs, manipulation, counseling concepts, and body movement, and combined them into a system that he called "polarity." The feeling of lightness and balance derived from polarity sessions brings constant affirmation of his positive use of internal energy and electromagnetic theory.

A polarity practitioner analyzes the magnetic current and its patterns of movement, and utilizes polarity's bodywork techniques to release energy blockages.

The term "polarity" comes from the fact that there are two sides, or poles, to everything in the universe: sun and moon, inhaling and exhaling, male energy and female energy, negative and positive electrical charges. Just as these energies in the universe must be balanced for life to continue, polarity seeks to balance the body's vital energy. The polarity system uses a four-part program to restore the body's proper energy balance.

Clear thinking is the basis of good health. According to polarity theory, a positive mental attitude occurs when people place no limitations on themselves and accept their emotions and abilities. Rather than resisting or repressing their intuition, clear-thinking people allow themselves and others to act freely.

Bodywork is used to balance the flow of energy and to sedate or tonify the organs. Polarity therapy links the body's inner dynamic energy centers (called *chakras,* the energy centers that are the source of all balance, in Sanskrit) by applying gentle pressure to sensitive contact points. Pressure is systematically applied on two points with both hands. This restores the body's subtle energy flow and rhythm. Thus balance, vitality, clarity, and well-being are restored. Polarity alleviates the energy blockages that are the root cause of disharmony, tension, pain, and structural distortions.

Body movement, known as polarity yoga or polarity energetics, is a series of easy stretching postures combining movement, breathing, and sound. These exercises increase vitality and they are easily integrated into daily life. Self-manipulations based on polarity techniques are also used.

Diet in polarity therapy emphasizes the use of fresh vegetables, fruits, and natural foods. However, the polarity practitioner always takes into account the individual's biochemical, social, and cultural patterns when making food recommendations. Individuals using the polarity approach are counseled, also, on how their emotions may affect eating and digestion.

The most important element of the polarity system is the practitioner's care and understanding of the client. The polarity practitioner is concerned with listening to the client's specific needs and responding to them in a way that is respectful, compassionate, and nonjudgmental. The polarity practitioner is a channel that a client uses to uncover his or her own self-healing powers.

Much of the popularity of polarity in the United States is due to the extensive teaching of the technique that takes place across the country, much of which was initiated by Dr. Stone's successor, Pierre Pennetier. Dr. Stone died in December 1981.

Naprapathy

For the past seventy-five years Chicago has harbored one of the best-kept secrets in the manipulative arts. Founded in 1907 by the young chiropractor Oakley Smith, the Chicago National College of Naprapathy continues today as the only school of naprapathy in the country. Naprapathy (nuh-PRAH-pathy) traces its geneaology from osteopathy (1875) through chiropractic (1895). The system integrates professional training with extensive anatomical research and with research of folk systems of manipulation to develop a gentle, unforced system of spinal and joint manipulation. Smith also developed a unique system of symbols and charts with which to record both the location and severity of body tensions and soreness as well as the specific corrective manipulation delivered.

Naprapaths assume that the body is inherently designed to function smoothly and efficiently. But contraction and rigidity of the soft connective tissues—muscles, tendons, and especially ligaments—can interfere with normal neurological and circulatory functioning. This interference occurs from the accumulation of major and minor injuries as well as postural, dietary, and psychogenic stress in the body's network of connective tissues. These injuries reduce the body's normal motion and resiliency. In response, naprapaths serve as practitioners of therapeutic manipulation who, with their trained touch, locate connective tissue contraction, and by gently stretching the tissues at these points of contraction, they restore structural and functional integrity. Naprapaths focus primarily upon the ligaments encasing the spinal column, where the connective tissues can so intimately affect the functioning of the spinal nerves, but they also work on other parts of the body.

When you visit a naprapath, he or she will first ask questions about your health history, including any present difficulties and your work and dietary habits, in order to establish primary areas of concern. But the substance of a naprapathic session occurs in the manipulative treatment as the naprapath starts to gently probe and push with the hands to test for resistance in the soft connective tissues as well as your response of soreness or pain to the palpation. From this information, the naprapath then systematically proceeds with rhythmic and repetitive "directos" (manipulative thrusts) in order to gently stretch contracted and painful areas. Treatments are usually experienced as comfortable and relaxing, even when the client has been experiencing acute pain. And once the tension is released, irritation to the nerves and areas of circulatory congestion return to more normal functioning. In conjunction, the naprapath will often suggest more healthful dietary, postural, and exercise patterns. After the initial session appointments generally last thirty minutes.

The college is recognized and chartered by the State of Illinois. And while at present the profession is not licensed nor is the school accredited, the profession is presently pursuing both. Several hundred naprapaths practice in the Chicago area with about 100 others spread throughout the country. And since 1970 a Swedish school of naprapathy has been flourishing in Stockholm and enjoys cooperation from the medical profession to further research naprapathic principles and technique.

Physiotherapy

Though this system draws its origins from Swedish massage, therapeutic gymnastics, and hydrotherapy, it has become more and more dominated by machinery. The object is still basically the same. The practitioner, with the use of various types of machinery, compels the body to act the way it might under normal stresses if there were no injury. The majority of physical therapists work in specialized physical therapy departments in hospitals or in rehabilitative medical centers. Many physical therapists in the past had virtually no massage training at all and used various mechanical and electrical apparatus to obtain the desired effects. The trend has been very slow, but some schools (usually associated with medical sschools) have begun minimal training classes in manipulation, shiatsu, and sports medicine. Many physical therapists have begun to open private offices, but they may still only see clients who are prescribed physical therapy by a physician. Though they are highly skilled practitioners, most problems handled by physical therapists can be corrected equally well by hands-on work—including therapeutic massage and postural correction—or by visualization or hydrotherapy.

Myotherapy (or Bonnie Prudden Technique)

Myotherapy was developed by Bonnie Prudden, who had previously developed her own exercise system. The technique works on the premise that most muscular pains have a trigger point which causes the muscle to go into spasm. Pressure on a trigger point causes the muscle spasm to relax and the pain to lessen or disappear. Fingers, knuckles and elbows are used to apply pressure, depending on the amount of pressure needed and the location of the trigger point. The technique also uses exercises to stretch the offending muscles, and cold water or ice is used on the muscle after a session. Often a problem may clear up after one session, but sometimes several sessions may be required.

Myotherapy is effective for a variety of problems, including lower back pain, tennis elbow, multiple sclerosis, bursitis, and headaches. Many of these problems may have roots in old injuries or falls which flare up when tensions arise later on in life.

The do-it-yourself approach is stressed, and both children and adults are able to learn simple trigger point techniques to relieve chronic and acute pains.

Muscular Therapy

This technique is the outgrowth of the work of Ben Benjamin, PhD, a dancer and student of movement theory. The Benjamin system is an integration of massage and education in movement. It is particularly attractive to dancers, though not limited to them. Included in the system are deep massage treatments, postural alignment, re-education in movement, and tension release exercises. Much of the movement work draws its philosophy from the writings of Mable Todd, Lulu Sweigard and Irmgard Bartinieff, all of whom helped foster a greater understanding of body mechanics and energy function. Muscular Therapy has its strongest value in pinpointing the effects of misalignment caused by improper use of the body in relation to gravity and in recognizing the effects of emotional repression in causing postural problems. In this sense it has some philosophical links to Alexander technique, Reichian Therapy, and Bioenergetics. By reducing tension, Muscular Therapy attempts to keep the body aligned, relaxed and healthy.

Ice Massage

This is a technique used by many different massage systems from a variety of cultures. Though commonly known for its value in first aid, few people are aware of the value of ice in sports medicine and massage. Ice massage will reduce pain and swelling, thereby increasing the healing environment so that the body may repair damaged tissue and increase the growth of normal healthy tissue. It may be used to increase circulation as it initially causes the surface blood vessels to contract. They will dilate upon completion of the ice massage. Ice massage is contraindicated for those individuals who have limited sensory nerve function and/or circulatory problems (e.g., diabetics). Ice massage may be used along the course of a nerve or directly on the sight of an injury. Using the technique properly involves skill and sensitivity. If used improperly, sensitive or injured tissue can become more damaged.

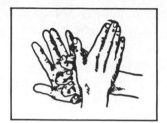

CHAPTER 2

ANATOMY AND PHYSIOLOGY

A basic knowledge of how the human body is constructed and operates is important for a full understanding of the therapeutic effects of any massage method. This understanding is part of being a well informed consumer or practitioner.

The human body is a miraculous instrument that most of us fail to fully appreciate or think much about until something goes wrong. While going about your daily routine, you probably take for granted the wonders that are involved every time you move. Whether you are doing something relatively simple like walking or something complex like typing or carpentry or playing basketball, each action involves an intricate chain of responses that would boggle your mind if you could actually view them. As you explore the subjects presented in this book, you will gain an understanding of how your body works and how massage can maintain and enhance your health and well being. You will find yourself developing an awareness and control that will add a new and satisfying dimension to your life.

The basic components of the body are cells, tissues, organs, and organ systems. Cells form tissues, tissues form organs, organs form systems, and the many systems form the human body.

 # Cells

The smallest living unit of the body is the cell—the physical basis of all life. Cells vary in size and shape, and they perform a variety of tasks. The largest cell is the ovum, the female reproductive cell. When the body is functioning properly, the cells, except for those in the brain, reproduce themselves. This characteristic of cells is a fundamental aspect of the self-healing capacity of the body.

An important benefit of any massage system is the maintenance of healthy cells. The improved circulation that massage and all bodywork produce will increase the supply of essential nutrients to the cells and prevent the buildup of waste material.

Tissues

Groups of similar cells form specialized tissues intended to perform particular functions. The most important for our purposes are:

Bone tissue. Hard connective tissue containing calcium and phosphate. As we age, bone tissue loses these vital minerals and as a result becomes brittle and breaks easily.

Epithelial tissue. Membranes that form the covering for the body's internal organs.

Soft connective tissue. Supports and connects other tissues and body parts and provides insulation for the body. Tendons and ligaments are examples of soft connective tissue.

Muscle tissue. The most abundant tissue in the body, it is made up of tough fibers. Balancing the structure and function of muscle tissue—relieving tension, poor muscle tone, and fatigue—is a primary concern of most massage and bodywork systems.

Nerve fibers. These receive and transmit stimuli to and from the sense organs and the brain.

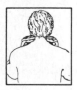

Organs

Just as cells form tissues, tissues form organs. Whereas similar cells join together to form tissue, organs are composed of several different kinds of tissue. The major organs are the skin, heart, kidneys, lungs, stomach, liver, gallbladder, spleen, and pancreas.

The largest, heaviest organ of the body is the skin, which measures about seventeen square feet on an average adult male. It is estimated that in one square inch of skin there are several million cells of various tissues, several feet of minute blood vessels, a dozen feet of nerve fibers, one hundred sweat glands, and just as many oil glands. The skin protects the body against injuries and parasitic invasions, regulates body temperature, aids in elimination of wastes, prevents too much loss of fluid from the body, stores food and water, receives sensations, and conducts vitamin D when exposed to the sun.

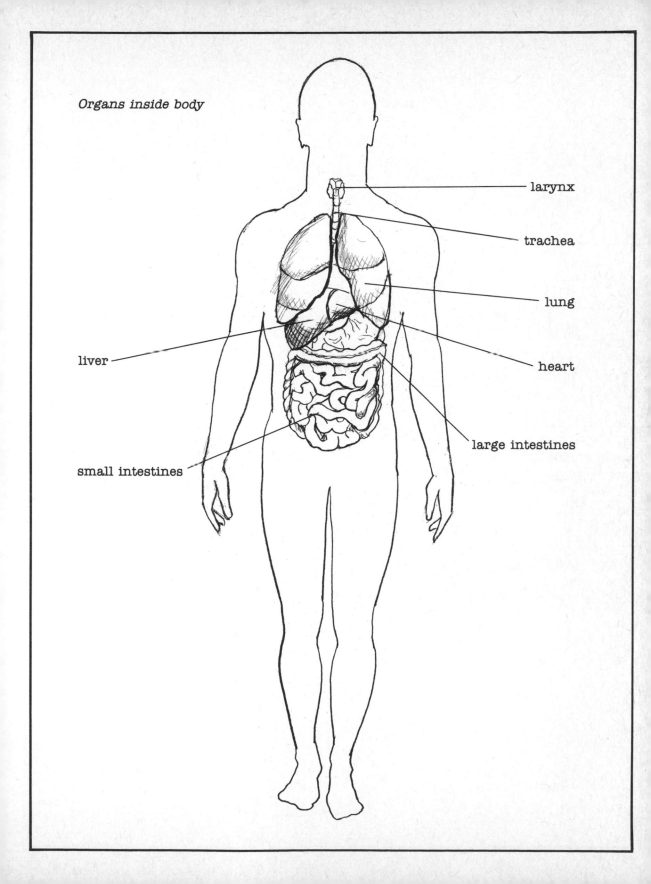

Organs inside body

larynx

trachea

lung

heart

liver

large intestines

small intestines

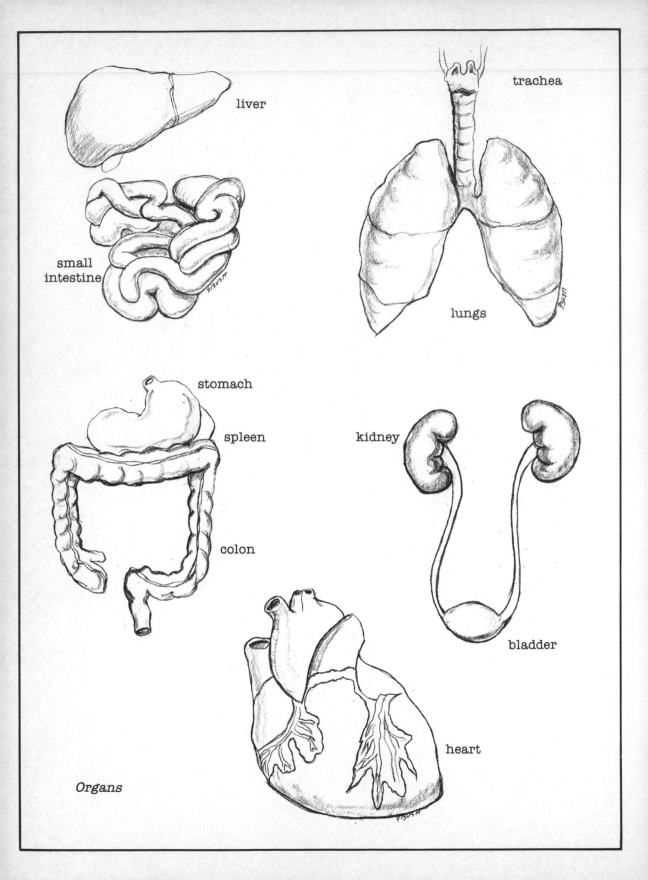

liver

trachea

small
intestine

lungs

stomach

spleen

kidney

colon

bladder

heart

Organs

The skin is composed of two distinct layers. The outer layer, or epidermis, consists of a number of layers of cells from which dry, dead cells are continually shed. The dermis, which lies beneath the epidermis, is considered a part of the skin. It contains nerve endings, capillaries, sweat glands, hair follicles, and sebaceous glands, which secrete the oily lubricant that maintains elasticity in the epidermis.

Disorders of the skin are numerous and include moles, small blood tumors, cancer, warts, blackheads, rashes due to allergy or infectious disease, hives, eczema, acne, boils, and ringworm. Although traditional Swedish massage, which involves quite a bit of rubbing and kneading of the skin, is generally contraindicated in many skin disorders, there are techniques described in chapter 3 that may be used without any complications.

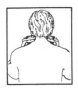

Systems

Organs join together with other organs and body parts to form systems. The human organism is an incredible collection of visible and invisible systems, each with a specialized task. An example is the digestive system, which includes the mouth, salivary glands, pharynx, esophagus, stomach, intestines, pancreas, liver, gallbladder, and appendix. Although there are many systems in the body, we will describe below only the skeletal, muscular, circulatory, nervous, respiratory, digestive, and urinary systems, because those are most readily affected by massage and body manipulation.

The Skeletal System

The skeletal system, which is composed primarily of bones and cartilage, provides support for the body in much the same way that a frame supports a house. Its two major functions are to protect the soft, easily damaged internal organs and to work together with the muscular system to provide the means for body movement and flexibility.

Bones are classified as either long, short, flat, or irregular. A general rule is that long and short bones are associated with movement and irregular and flat bones protect the internal organs. For example, the bones of the skull, which protect the brain, are flat; the femur and humerus, which are located in the leg and the arm respectively, are long bones. Skilled massage affects bones by balancing the muscles and tissues that determine their alignment and locomotion.

Cartilage is the soft connective tissue that covers the joints, between the bones. It is easily damaged and may be involved in diseases of the joints such as osteoarthritis.

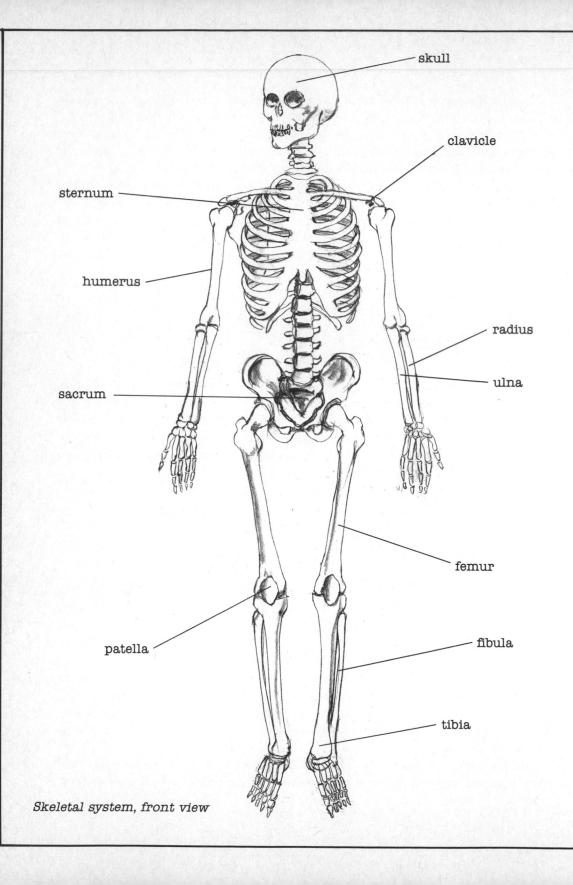

skull

clavicle

sternum

humerus

radius

ulna

sacrum

femur

patella

fibula

tibia

Skeletal system, front view

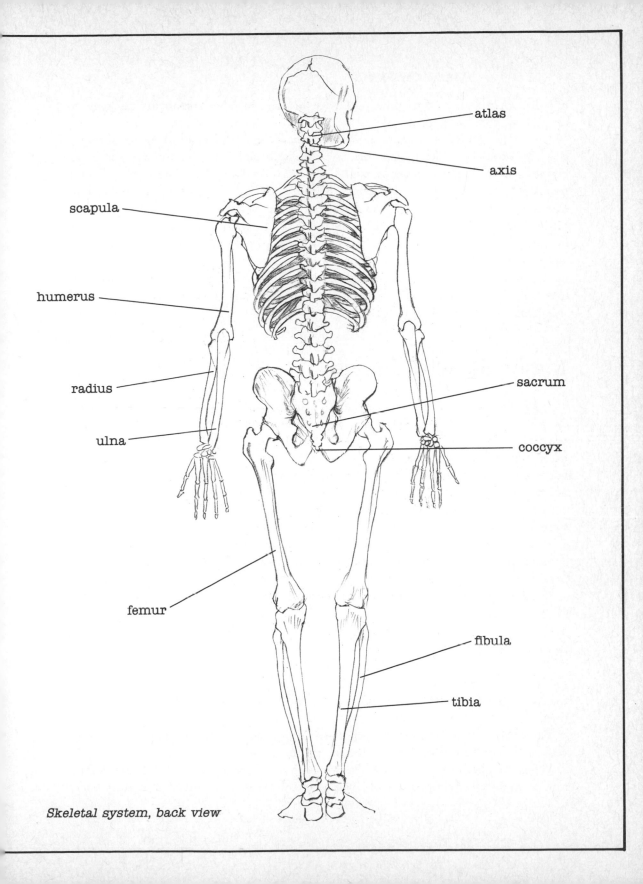

atlas

axis

scapula

humerus

radius

ulna

sacrum

coccyx

femur

fibula

tibia

Skeletal system, back view

Cartilages can tear or be damaged. Massage and certain water treatments can help to tonify and strengthen them.

Joints, the points of connection between the bones, are classified as immovable, slightly movable, or freely movable. The strength and flexibility of the joints are maintained by muscles, tendons, and ligaments. Tendons attach muscles to bones; ligaments attach bones to other bones. Quite a few of the joints in the body have extremely limited movement. One such joint is the sacroiliac, the joint in the pelvic girdle between the sacrum and the ilium. One of the many wonders of nature is that during pregnancy there is a relaxation of the strong ligaments that hold this joint in place, with a resultant spreading of the bones to allow for delivery. The freely movable joints, those most important to body movement, should be of primary concern in a good massage. Freely movable joints are the toes, fingers, ankles, wrists, knees, elbows, shoulders, neck, and hips.

Major Skeletal Bones

Skull. The bony framework of the head. It consists of eight cranial bones that protect the brain and fourteen facial bones that provide the contours of the face. Many bodywork systems, for example SOT, TMJ, and craniopathy, involve specific cranial manipulations, since their practitioners believe that imbalances of the cranial as well as the facial bones may result in health problems such as lower back pain, specific vision problems, neurological imbalances, sacral problems, and foot and respiratory imbalances.

Spinal column (backbone). The basic structure in the skeletal system and the major support for the head and trunk. It also protects the highly sensitive spinal cord, which carries nerve impulses to and from the brain and controls the activities of glands, organs, and muscles. Damage to the spinal cord is extremely serious and often results in paralysis in different parts of the body.

In adults the spinal column consists of twenty-six movable vertebrae; seven in the neck (cervical vertebrae); twelve in the upper back and chest (thoracic vertebrae); and five in the lower back (lumbar vertebrae). The other two movable vertebrae are the sacrum and the coccyx.

The first cervical vertebra connects with the occipital bone of the skull, which forms the back of the head. It is known as the atlas. The second cervical vertebra is known as the axis. The others are designated by their number down from the occipital bone (e.g., third cervical vertebra, fourth cervical vertebra, etc.).

The twelve thoracic vertebrae support the upper back and chest, and it is to these vertebrae that the twelve pairs of ribs are attached.

When we speak of the lower back, we are usually concerned with the five highly mobile lumbar vertebrae. Over one-half of the total body weight is carried by these

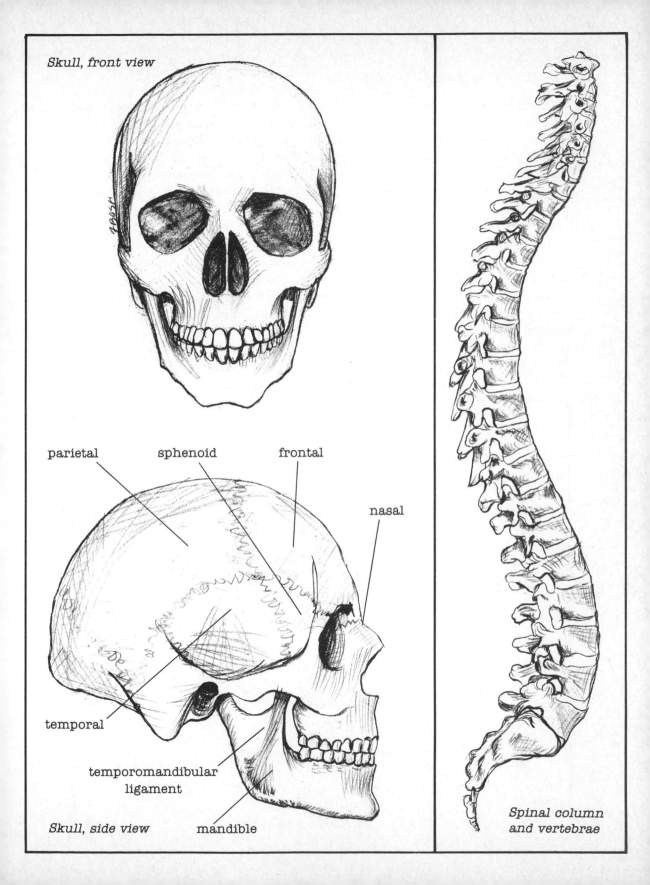

Skull, front view

parietal

sphenoid

frontal

nasal

temporal

temporomandibular
ligament

Skull, side view

mandible

*Spinal column
and vertebrae*

vertebrae before being passed down to the feet. In addition to the powerful lower-back muscles, the muscles of the abdomen, buttocks, and legs provide support and movement to the lower-back area. Nonetheless, this is a very vulnerable area which is subject to the stresses of poor walking and sitting habits. In addition, all too often people attempt to lift heavy objects by using the muscles in this area and as a consequence exert extreme pressure on it, sometimes causing the disks to rupture, creating an extremely serious health problem.

The sacrum is located between the fifth lumbar vertebrae and the coccyx. It appears to be one triangular shaped bone but is in fact five fused vertebrae. Many of the effects of posture are strongly indicated here since body weight is distributed to the hip joints by means of the sacrum's connection with the pelvic girdle.

The coccyx, sometimes called the tailbone, is a small triangular bone attached to the bottom of the sacrum. It consists of four tiny, fused vertebrae. Most traditional health professionals consider it to be functionally unimportant. However, both the sacrum and the coccyx, together with the pelvis, are major storage areas for vital life energy. Rapid

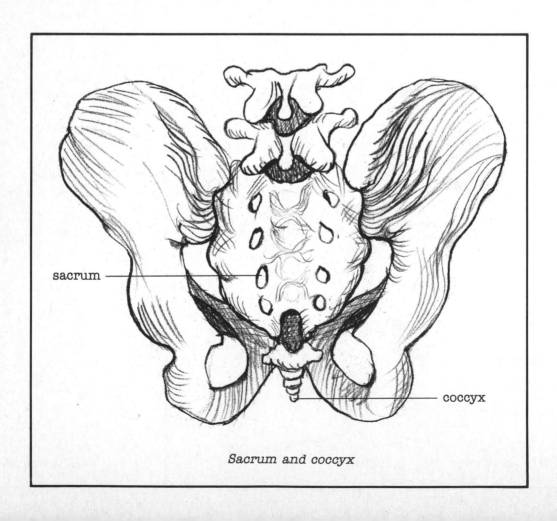

sacrum

coccyx

Sacrum and coccyx

energy balancing as well as structural changes may be brought about when body manipulation techniques are applied to these areas.

The entire spinal column is a major holding place for tension. Practitioners of some bodywork systems, such as chiropractic, osteopathy, and naprapathy, believe that imbalances in the spinal column are the major cause of health problems. Other systems acknowledge the importance of the spinal column, but their practitioners take a different approach. Chiropractic philosophy, for example, believes that correcting the position of the vertebrae will affect nerve and muscular functioning. We believe that in many situations of spinal imbalance, stabilizing the muscles will cause the vertebrae to correct themselves. There are exercise systems that will have a similar effect. There are without a doubt certain situations, such as back problems, and migraine headaches, where chiropractic or osteopathic manipulations work much more efficiently. But this is not always the case. It is for this reason that many chiropractors have begun using additional body manipulation techniques, particularly kinesiology.

Clavicle (collar bone). A straight bone joined to the sternum (breastbone) at its inner end and to the scapula (shoulder blade) at its outer end. Because the clavicle is fragile and cannot endure heavy pressure, special care should be taken when doing bodywork around it.

Ribs. Protect the lungs and other essential areas in the chest. At the end of each of the twenty-four ribs is cartilage, which, in the first seven pairs connects to the sternum (breastbone). If this cartilage tears or is damaged, or if the ribs are moved, massage and body manipulation may prove to be valuable. Rib pairs eight through ten are connected to one another by a continuous cartilage but do not attach to the breastbone. Rib pairs eleven and twelve are called "floating ribs" and have no attachment other than to the thoracic vertebrae.

The muscles of the chest cavity (the thoracic wall) are essential for breathing. Although the diaphragm is the most important muscle involved in inhalation, the muscles between the ribs also play an important role.

Sternum (breastbone). A flat bone in the chest area that is attached to and stabilizes the ribs. Fractures of this bone generally heal without trouble, but it is wise to use caution when doing massage and bodywork in this area since the heart lies directly behind it.

Scapula (shoulder blade). A triangular-shaped pair of bones in the upper portion of the back on either side of the thoracic vertebrae. Each is about the size of a hand. Most of the bone is very thin, but the outer border is rounded and strong and embedded in powerful muscles. Because they are well padded, they are not often broken.

Tightness of the muscles along the insides of the scapula generally indicates imbalance in the respiratory or digestive system. Relaxing these muscles through the techniques mentioned in chapter 3 will relieve many problems associated with digestion and respiration.

Pelvis. The pelvis is a large pair of bones that are located near the center of the body.

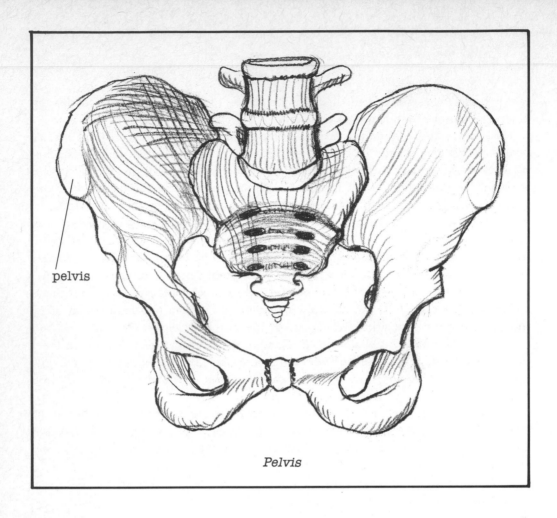

pelvis

Pelvis

The pelvis acts as an attachment for the spine, sacrum, and femur (upper leg bone). It acts as an anchor; the body pivots around it and its weight is balanced on the pelvis. Although pelvic injuries can leave you temporarily immobilized, problems can often be corrected through rest and body manipulation to bring about postural alignment.

Humerus. A major skeletal bone located in the upper arm. At the shoulder it fits into a shallow socket in the scapula and forms the shoulder joint. This bone often is dislocated from the shoulder socket. Breaks are common, but will heal once the bone is set. When massaging the areas around a healed bone, keep in mind that the muscles may be weak, because they have not been used as much as those around the arm that is not broken.

Ulna and Radius. The two bones of the forearm. The ulna is the longer and thinner of the two and forms the bony projection at the elbow. At the wrist, the strain falls on the radius. When one of these bones is broken, the other is usually affected.

Carpals. The eight bones that form the wrist. These bones are connected to the metacarpals, which are later connected to the phalanges. Surrounding muscles and tissue often need massaging because they can cause pain and stiffness at the joints.

Metacarpals. The five bones that lie between the wrist and fingers.

44

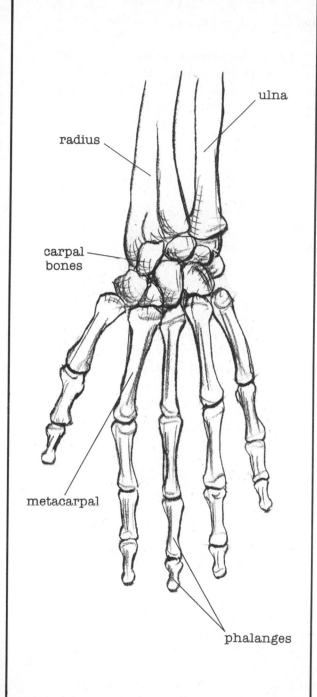

radius

ulna

carpal
bones

metacarpal

phalanges

Bones in wrist and hand

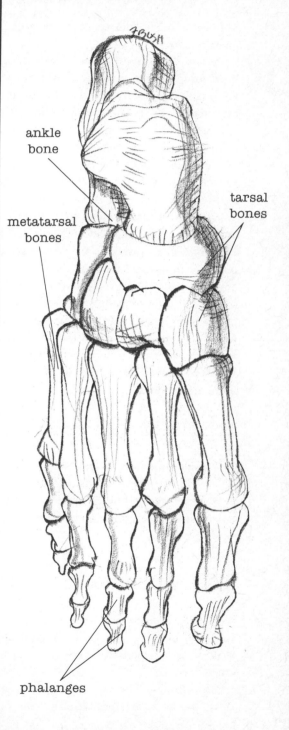

ankle
bone

metatarsal
bones

tarsal
bones

phalanges

Bones in ankle and foot

Phalanges. The fourteen bones on each hand that form the fingers and on each foot that form the toes.

Femur. The longest bone in the body and the only bone between the hip joint and the knee joint. The top of the femur breaks easily when fallen upon and is particularly vulnerable in elderly people. Increasing fragility of the bones as people age is often exacerbated by poor dietary habits. Weakening of the bones is also caused by osteoporosis, which often results from the use of cortisone to produce symptomatic relief from osteoarthritis and other health problems.

Fibula and Tibia. The two bones between the knee and the ankle. The tibia, which is known as the shinbone, is the larger of the two. The fibula anchors the lower part of the body to the ankle and is easily broken.

Tarsals. The seven bones that form the ankle. As in the carpals or wrists, the muscles around this joint may become stiff and blockages may impede the blood flow. These blockages can cause pain or discomfort that can be helped by the massage techniques outlined in chapter four.

Metatarsals. The five bones that form the metatarsal arch and the ball of the foot.

Most of the imbalances that take place in the feet are the result of the pull of gravity on body weight. However, improper posture as well as poorly fitted shoes are also the cause of many problems in this area. In proper posture, body weight is spread equally between both feet. The majority of this weight is borne by the heel bone (calcaneus), with the remainder resting on the outer weightbearing arch of the foot and associated metatarsal bones.

Benefits of massage for the skeletal system

- maintains posture and body balance
- reduces muscular tension that eventually causes structural problems
- increases the flow of nutrients to the bones
- promotes elimination of waste matter

The Muscular System

Muscles are the most abundant tissues in the body and comprise at least two-fifths of the total body weight. They contain blood vessels and nerves. Their primary responsibility is to facilitate body movement. This is made possible by the following characteristics:

Contractility. The capacity to shrink or contract that is inherent in all cells. Muscle cells, however, are specialized to contract, but only in length, not width.

Extensibility. The capacity to stretch. After a muscle has been stretched it contracts much more strongly than before. This is why stretching exercises are so important to the health of your muscles.

Irritability. The capacity to respond to stimuli. If chemicals, heat, electrical shock, or pressure are applied to muscles, they will contract.

Elasticity. The capacity to convey an impulse. When a muscle contracts, the fibers become tense and pull the bones together, resulting in movement. If a muscle has difficulty contracting, it may be either flaccid or fatigued. Flaccidity in a muscle is caused by non-use. Fatigue is caused by excessive use, resulting in a depletion of oxygen resources in the muscle and a buildup of a waste product known as lactic acid.

In body manipulation is it important to keep in mind that muscles usually act in groups and that any given movement is the result of several muscles working together. Muscles move the bones or body parts located immediately above or below them. For example, muscles in the neck move the head; muscles in the thigh move the lower leg.

The expansive and contractive properties of muscles also help to produce body heat as well as to determine the body's form and posture. A person who has good posture will often seem highly charismatic regardless of other physical characteristics; a physically beautiful person with poor posture may seem less attractive.

There are many muscles that will need attention at one time or another because of excess tension flaccidity, or fatigue. The ones shown in figure 12 are those that are most often manipulated or massaged in order to maintain body flexibiliy, vitality, harmony, and balance.

The terms below are used to describe muscles based on the kind of movement they produce:

Flexor:	Bends a body part.
Extensor:	Extends a body part.
Adductor:	Draws a body part toward the midline.
Abductor:	Draws a body part away from the midline.
Rotator:	Revolves a body part on its axis.
Levator:	Raises a body part.
Depressor:	Lowers a body part.
Sphincter:	Closes or reduces the size of an opening.
Tensor:	Makes a body part tense or more rigid.
Supinator:	Turns the hand palm upward.
Pronator:	Turns the hand palm downward.

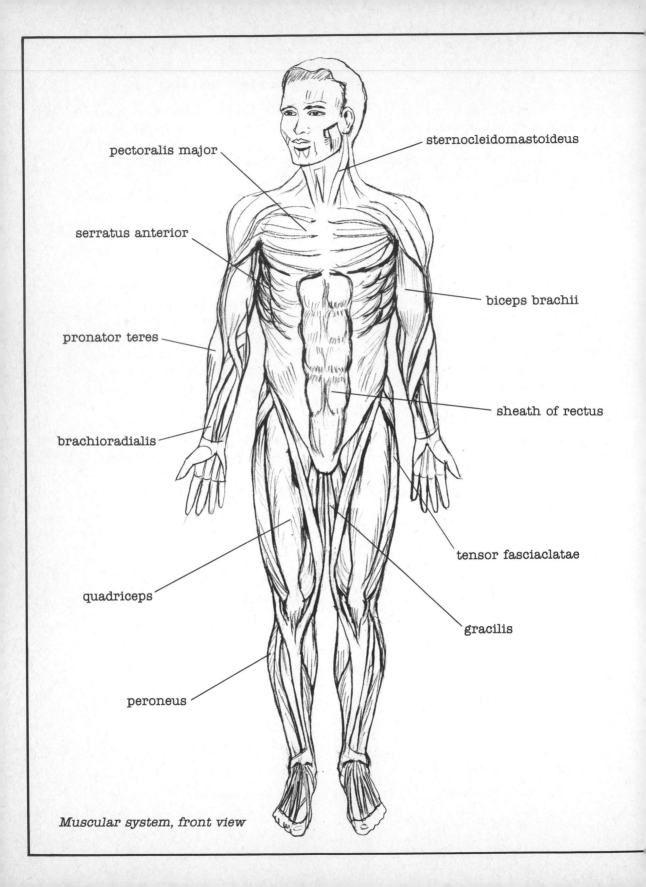

pectoralis major

sternocleidomastoideus

serratus anterior

biceps brachii

pronator teres

sheath of rectus

brachioradialis

tensor fasciaclatae

quadriceps

gracilis

peroneus

Muscular system, front view

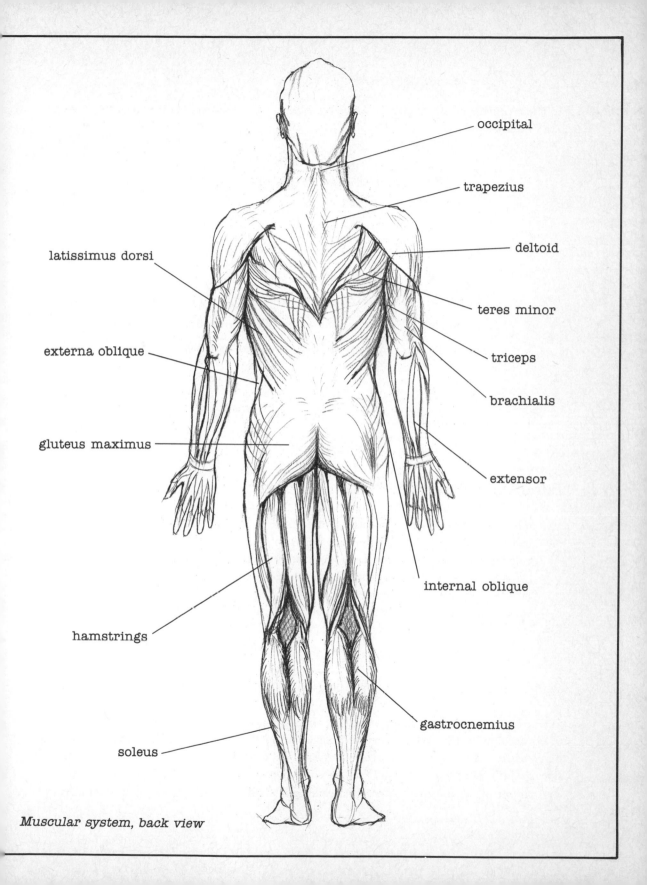

occipital

trapezius

deltoid

latissimus dorsi

teres minor

triceps

externa oblique

brachialis

gluteus maximus

extensor

internal oblique

hamstrings

gastrocnemius

soleus

Muscular system, back view

The terms below are used to describe positions of the body and are useful in locating parts or imbalances:

Anatomic Position:	Facing the observer with palms turned forward.
Superior:	Toward the head.
Inferior:	Toward the feet.
Posterior:	Toward the back of the body.
Anterior:	Toward the front of the body.
Medial:	Down the center of the body, going from head to foot.
Lateral:	Across the body, going from the midline to the outside.
Median:	Across the body, going from the outside to the midline.
Exterior:	On the surface of the body.
Interior:	Inside the body.
Proximal:	Nearer to the joint of attachment.
Distal:	Farther from the point of attachment.

Benefits of massage for the muscular system

O relieves muscle tension and relaxes muscle spasm
O increases the supply of blood and nutrients to muscles
O helps to eliminate waste matter from muscles (especially lactic acid)
O helps restore tone to flaccid muscles and partially compensates for lack of exercise and inactivity because of illness or injury
O eliminates or prevents muscle adhesions resulting from injury
O increases flexibility and strength of joints

The Circulatory System

The circulatory system transports blood and lymph, a fluid that aids in the production of white blood cells, throughout the body. During this process it carries oxygen and nutrients to all the body cells, removes wastes, protects the body from disease, aids in the regulation of body heat, and energizes the body.

A circuitlike arrangement of arteries, veins, and capillaries feeds blood to all the parts

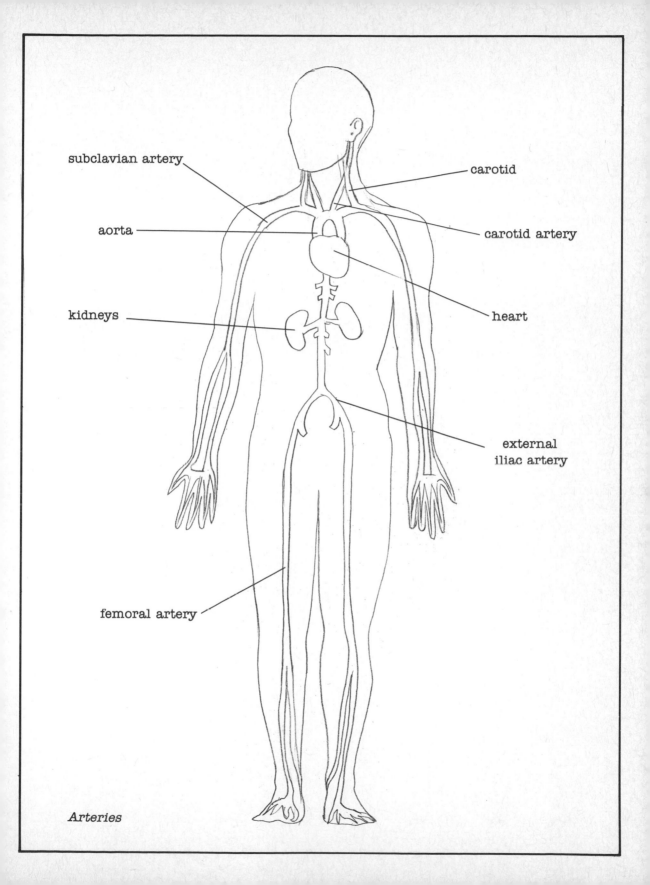

subclavian artery

carotid

aorta

carotid artery

heart

kidneys

external
iliac artery

femoral artery

Arteries

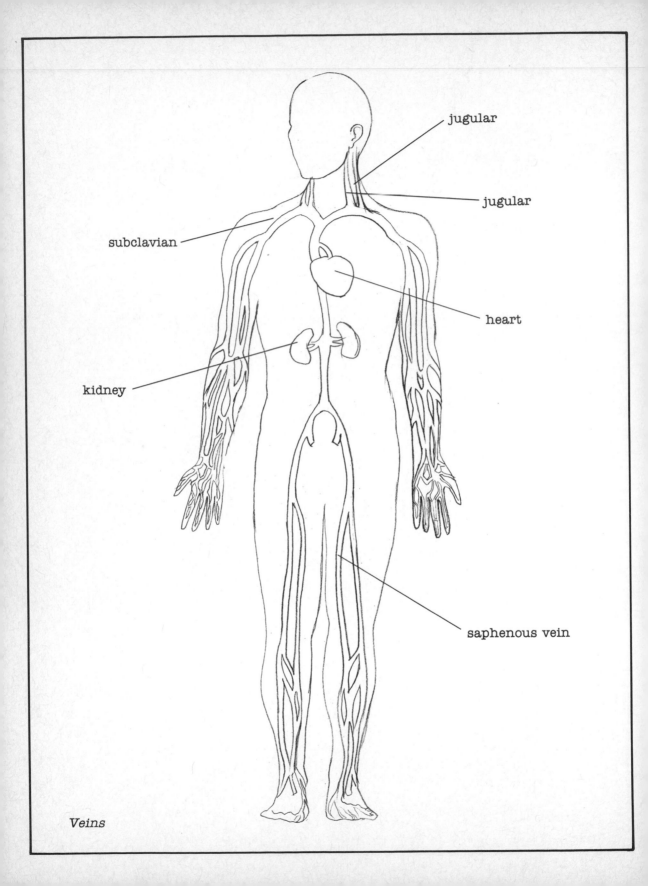

jugular

jugular

subclavian

heart

kidney

saphenous vein

Veins

of the body. The starting point is the heart. Arteries carry blood away from the heart; veins carry blood to the heart. By contraction of its muscular walls, the heart forces oxygenated blood out of the left ventricle, through the aortic valves and into the aorta, from which other arteries branch out into the body. The smallest branches of the arteries end in small blood vessels called capillaries, which in turn end in veins. These veins finally merge to form the *inferior vena cava* and *superior vena cava,* which return deoxygenated blood to the right auricle of the heart from the trunk, legs, head, neck, and arms.

By the contraction of the right ventricle, blood is then forced through the pulmonary valves into the pulmonary arteries, which carry blood to and from the lungs. In the lungs, carbon dioxide is eliminated from the blood and oxygen is secured. The oxygenated blood then returns through the pulmonary veins to the left auricle of the heart and then passes through the bicuspid valve into the left ventricle, which again sends it into the aorta, to start the process again.

Lymph is a slightly yellow fluid that aids in the production of white blood cells, which in turn strengthen the immune system and help combat infections. This fluid is derived chiefly from blood plasma that filters through the capillary walls into spaces between the cells. It is then drained by lymph capillaries and circulated through the body by a network of small vessels or channels.

Accumulations of lymphatic tissue found at intervals throughout the body in such locations as the armpit, neck, groin, abdomen, and chest area are called lymph nodes. These nodes serve as filters to keep waste particles, especially bacteria, from entering the bloodstream. They become inflamed and swollen and are easily palpable.

The movement of lymph depends on the contraction of muscles. Consequently, immobility due to pain or paralysis seriously interferes with lymph drainage. There are lymph nodes throughout the body. When these nodes become inflamed or swollen there can be a structural cause such as carrying a heavy bag constantly on one shoulder. This will cause the lymph nodes under the arm to become imbalanced. Check before you massage such areas, since it is possible to increase the swelling. However, if it is indicated, massage to this area can be soothing, and help the blocked gland to open up, allowing the lymph to flow freely.

Benefits of massage for the circulatory system

- ○ improves blood circulation and relieves congestion
- ○ increases supply of oxygen and nutrients to cells throughout the body
- ○ eases the strain on the heart by helping to return blood to this vital organ, especially in cases of forced inactivity due to illness or injury
- ○ pushes the movement of lymph through the body, thereby strengthening the immune system and eliminating toxic wastes.

The Nervous System

The nervous system is the body's control center—it regulates and coordinates all other systems and organs. It consists of a highly developed central nervous system, which includes the brain and spinal cord, and the autonomic nervous system, consisting of nerves and groups of nerve cells.

The basic unit in the nervous system is the nerve cell (neuron), which conducts electrochemical energy forms known as nerve impulses. *Sensory nerve cells* carry these impulses to the brain from the sense organs—the skin, eyes, ear, nose, and taste buds. *Motor nerve cells* carry impulses from the brain to the muscles. When you touch, see, hear, smell, or taste, it is the result of sensory nerves transmitting impulses to the brain. When you respond to a stimulus or you move your body, it is because the motor nerves are now carrying messages from the brain.

The central nervous system acts as a force to generate energy, movement and thought. The messages that it sends out tell the body what to do. Often there is a loose connection between the mind and the body, leading to conditions, such as cerebral palsy, in which the body cannot be controlled by the mind. Or, there are cases where the reverse occurs, and the mind does not function and cannot send signals to the body. When this occurs, the muscles may have a tendency to be spasmic and uncontrolled. Massage to these areas can relax and help to train them to be controlled.

Massage can be used to relax the nerves or in the case of someone who may be sluggish and mentally drowsy, a tonifying massage can perk up the entire system. The nervous system stimulates and triggers the emotions.

Important parts of the nervous system

Cerebrum. The largest structure of the brain. It controls conscious, voluntary processes.

Cerebral Cortex. A gray tissue that forms the outer layer of the cerebrum. It is responsible for many higher functions such as talking, thinking, memory, and judgment.

Cerebellum. The section of the brain behind and below the cerebrum. It is responsible for the coordination of complex muscular movements such as typing, dancing, and athletics.

Thalamus. A large mass of gray tissue located at the base of the brain. It sends sensory stimuli to the cerebral cortex and interprets them. The thalamus also appears to be involved in emotional responses and the integration of speech.

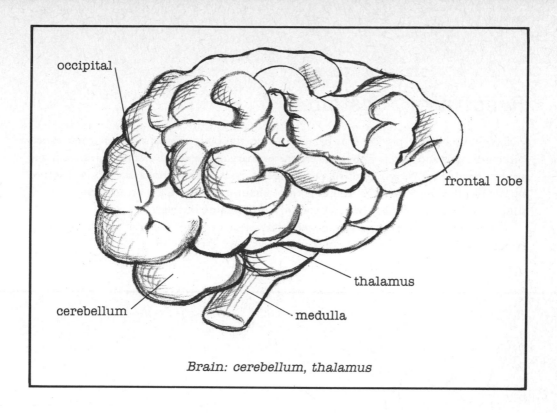

occipital

frontal lobe

thalamus

cerebellum

medulla

Brain: cerebellum, thalamus

Hypothalamus. Lies below the thalamus. It helps regulate body temperature, water balance, sugar and fat metabolism, and the secretions of the endocrine glands.

Spinal Cord. A column of nerve tissue beginning in the brain and ending at the second lumbar vertebra. All nerves to the trunk and limbs pass out of the spinal cord, the center for reflex actions.

The *autonomic nervous system* is generally concerned with the control of unconscious and involuntary body functions. It regulates the glands, the heart muscle, and smooth muscle tissue such as that found in the walls of the digestive organs and blood vessels. It is divided into two sections: the sympathetic and the parasympathetic. The *sympathetic* nervous system controls responses to stressful situations by engaging what are commonly known as "fight or flight" reactions. These include increased heart and respiratory rates, sweating, dilation of the pupils, and increased flow of blood to the skeletal muscles. The *parasympathetic* system controls normal body functions such as digestion, absorption of nutrients, draining of the urinary bladder, and the reduction of heart and respiration rates.

Benefits of massage for the nervous system

- can either sedate or stimulate the nervous system, depending on the technique used
- by balancing the nervous system, affects all the systems of the body

Respiratory System

Respiration is the process that brings air into the body, absorbs oxygen, and expels carbon dioxide and water. The lungs are the primary organ in the respiratory system and are responsible for carrying out this exchange of gases. In the lungs oxygen is absorbed by the blood, which then distributes it throughout the body. Each breath brings a fresh supply of air to the lungs, but some air always remains in them.

The respiratory system consists of the nasal passages (nose), pharynx (throat), larynx (voice box), trachea (windpipe), bronchi, lungs, and diaphragm.

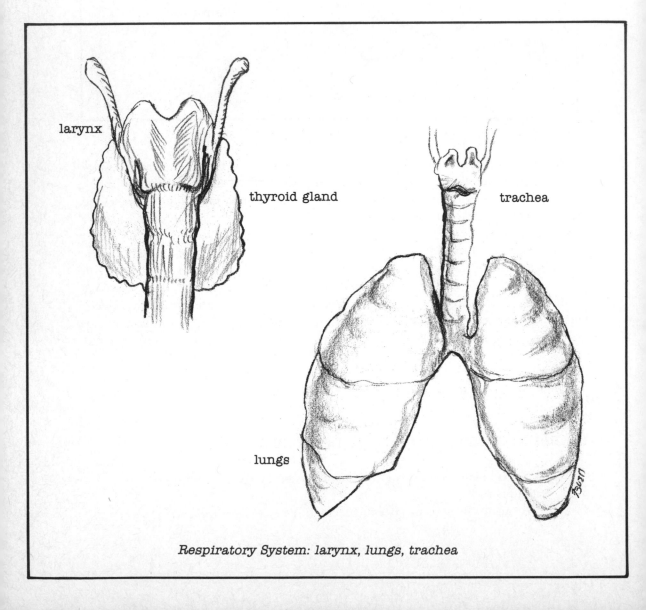

Respiratory System: larynx, lungs, trachea

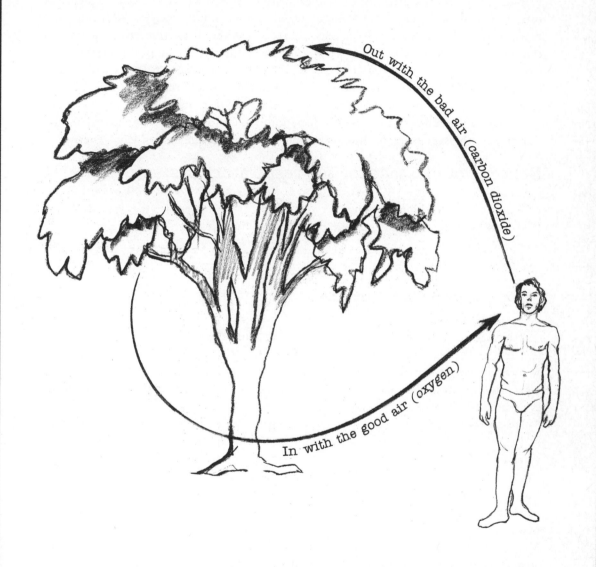

Out with the bad air (carbon dioxide)

In with the good air (oxygen)

Photosynthesis

The muscles of the chest cavity (the thoracic wall) are essential for breathing. The diaphragm is the most important muscle involved in breathing, but the intercostal muscles (the ones between the ribs) also play an important role. When you inhale, your diaphragm lowers and your ribs rise. In exhalation the reverse occurs. This sequence of inhalation and exhalation occurs about eighteen times a minute when the body is at rest. During this process, the expansion and contraction of the diaphragm creates a rhythm that affects the entire organism biochemically, structurally, and most especially, emotionally. As a result, increased efficiency and balance in breathing patterns will greatly affect your mental, emotional, and physical wellbeing. When massage is utilized, the respiratory system can be given a chance to open up and clear itself. Often the trachea or the lungs can be blocked by particles that inhibit the proper action of the system. By clearing it, massage helps breathing become stronger and the system gains energy.

Benefits of massage for the respiratory system

○ improves breathing patterns
○ aids in relief of many long-term respiratory difficulties such as asthma and bronchitis

The Digestive System

The digestive system alters the physical and chemical form of food so that it can be utilized by the body for energy and cell restoration. The digestive system includes the mouth, salivary glands, pharynx, esophagus, stomach, large and small intestines, pancreas, liver, gallbladder, and appendix. These organs form a tube that runs through the system and is known as the alimentary canal.

Food passes from the mouth, where it is prepared for digestion, through the pharynx and esophagus to the stomach, where it undergoes the early stages of digestion. Within three to four hours of eating, the stomach is empty and digestion continues in the small intestine by means of bile, which is secreted by the liver, pancreatic juice, and intestinal juice.

Many people believe that the liver, responsible for purifying the body and producing new cells, ranks in importance with the heart in ensuring a strong, healthy body. Massaging the internal organs can relieve gas and in some cases even soothe pain in this area. Massaging the colon and the stomach will also aid in digestive disorders.

Benefits of massage for the digestive system

○ improves the function of the liver

○ acts as a mechanical cleanser, pushing out waste products, particularly in those who suffer from constipation
○ relieves spastic colon

The Urinary System

The elimination of waste from the body is the main function of the urinary system, whose principal organs are the kidneys, ureters, bladder, and urethra. Urine is secreted by the kidneys through the ureters to the bladder, stored in the bladder, and then is discharged through the urethra. Urine analysis can aid in detecting diseases of the kidney and other parts of the urinary tract, as well as in the diagnosis of diabetes.

The kidneys are important in regulating blood pressure as well as in maintaining the body's water balance. At least one kidney must function in order for life to be sustained.

Benefits of massage for the urinary system

○ massaging the kidneys can cleanse the blood and tonify the entire system
○ in problems of swelling in the body, massage can affect the elimination of fluids

You do not have to know a great deal about anatomy and physiology to give a good "home" massage—certainly not to be an informed consumer of massage—but when body manipulation is used for even the most basic therapeutic purposes, such as releasing tight muscles or relieving tension, a general understanding of how the body works and how massage affects the body's various organs and systems will help you in several important ways. First, you will be better able to gauge when *not* to massage or be massaged (this is discussed in chapter 3). Second, you can begin to relate common physical symptoms to particular body manipulation therapies that may be helpful. Most important, an understanding of how your body works will aid you in your overall health regimen.

Massage should be an important part of that regimen, so do not get so bogged down trying to remember the cells, tissues, organs, and systems that you forget that massage is art as well as science. The essence of any body manipulation system is hands-on, communicative contact.

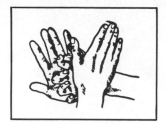

CHAPTER 3

MASSAGE TECHNIQUES

If you are a massage consumer, that is, you pay to be massaged, you can choose a practitioner skilled in any of the more than a score of bodywork methods. But if you are like most people you turn to massage when you ache, are tense, or have minor muscular injuries. Your "masseur" or "masseuse" is your spouse, friend, coach, or teammate. But you want more than the sensual rub-down offered by most massage books, you want to use techniques that will relieve your ache, ease your tension, or help heal your sore muscles.

As massage practitioners, we wanted to offer all the possible benefits of body manipulation to our clients, yet we recognized the impracticality—and discomfort to our clients—of constantly changing from one technique to another. Drawing from many bodywork systems, we compiled a "short hand" of nine basic massage techniques that together offer a full range of therapeutic and pleasurable body manipulation.

Our nine techniques are intended to provide a simple, usable massage system for lay people and health care professionals. Though we believe this system rivals the best formal body manipulation systems in its practicality, simplicity, and therapeutic effects, it is not intended to substitute for the several dozen separate body manipulation systems and subsystems. Each has its particular benefits and shortcomings, its distinct effects, and its particular hands-on technique and philosophy. But most systems require years of training before one masters its techniques and realizes its distinct benefits. We believe massage can benefit everyone and that everyone, with a little time and a little more sensitivity, can learn to give a good therapeutic massage.

Each of these nine techniques is intended for use with specific problems, and all of them can be mastered with a bit of practice. Once they are learned, they can be used for

The nine
basic
massage
techniques

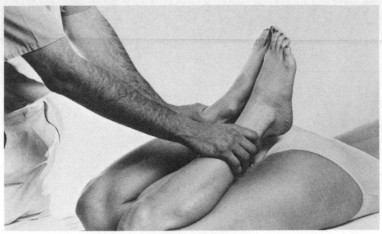

Range of Motion
(back knee bend)

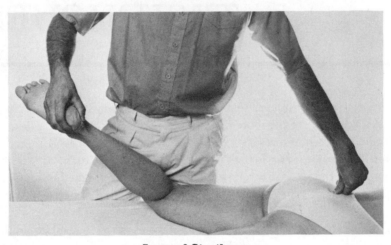

Law of Similars
(sacrum to heel)

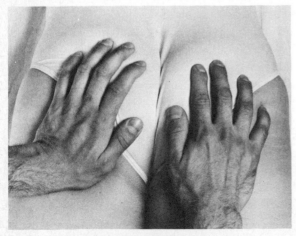

Muscle Squeeze
(on buttocks)

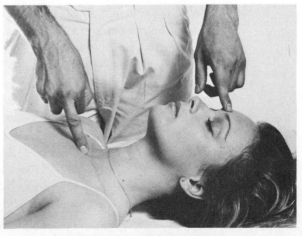

Vital Force Contact
(third eye and crest of sternum)

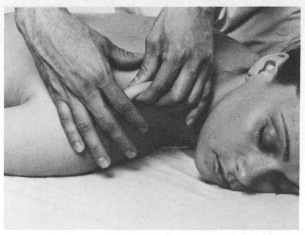

Kneading
(muscle kneading on shoulder)

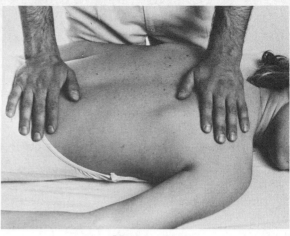

Muscle Rock
(on spine)

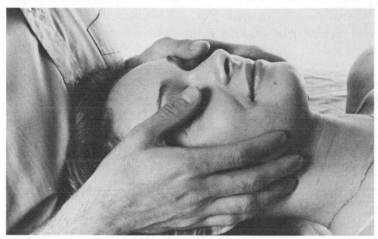

General Rhythmic Pressure
(on eyes)

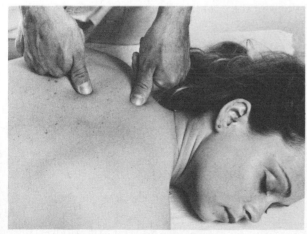

Circular Rhythmic Pressure
(on spine)

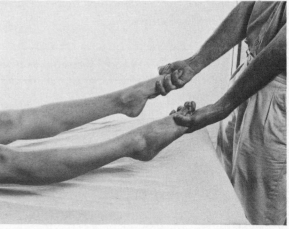

Pull and Stretch
(to legs)

a tremendous variety of ailments for which massage is needed, and for maintaining general health, comfort and vitality. All nine techniques can be used on oneself, although it is always helpful and more fun to work with a partner in learning how to massage. Massage is touch and touch is communication. Having someone communicate with as you learn massage will make it a more enriching experience.

Range of Motion

This is a gentle movement to help evaluate and improve flexibility in the joints. Each joint has a normal range of motion. You can evaluate the condition of the muscles associated with each joint by working it through its normal range of motion.

Step 1

Slowly try to rotate the joint through its normal range of motion, moving it in all ways possible. Hold the body part to be worked on in your hand to give it support as you move the joint through the normal range.

Step 2

Tightness or limitation in movement can sometimes be relieved by gently moving the joint through its range of motion. If not, apply Rhythmic Pressure in the area of blockage.

Step 3

Repeat gentle Range of Motion exercises periodically—about every two or three hours—until the tightness or limitation of movement is lessened. Slowly rotate the joint six times in one direction and then six times in the opposite direction. Repeat the cycle three times.

> ***Caution:*** *Stop the movement if there is intense pain. Never force the joint.*

Law of Similars

The Law of Similars is an extremely gentle technique. It is based on the concept that there is a reflex action between certain body parts. By placing one hand on the point of blockage and the second on its corresponding reflex point, the power of the body's healing energy is stimulated.

The number of Law of Similars reflex points runs into the hundreds. For simplicity and clarity, we are listing below only those reflex points that we use most often.

Superior Points	Inferior Points
Fingers	Toes
(each finger corresponds to a toe)	
Palm	Bottom of foot
Forearm	Shin
Elbow	Knee
Upper arm	Thigh
Inside border of shoulderblade	Calves
Inside border of shoulderblade	Buttocks
Buttocks	Calves
Occipital bone	Sacrum
Sacrum	Back of heel
Shoulder joint	Hip joint
Wrist	Ankle

Step 1

Place one hand over an area of discomfort and place your other hand over the corresponding reflex points. Simply lay your palms flat on your partner's body so that your entire hand is in contact with your partner's skin. Hold the contact for three to five minutes.

Step 2

If you want to be more specific, you may use your thumb or finger. The superior contact, the one closer to the head, should be made with the thumb or index finger. The inferior contact, the one farther from the head, should be made with the thumb or middle finger.

Body chart of law of similars

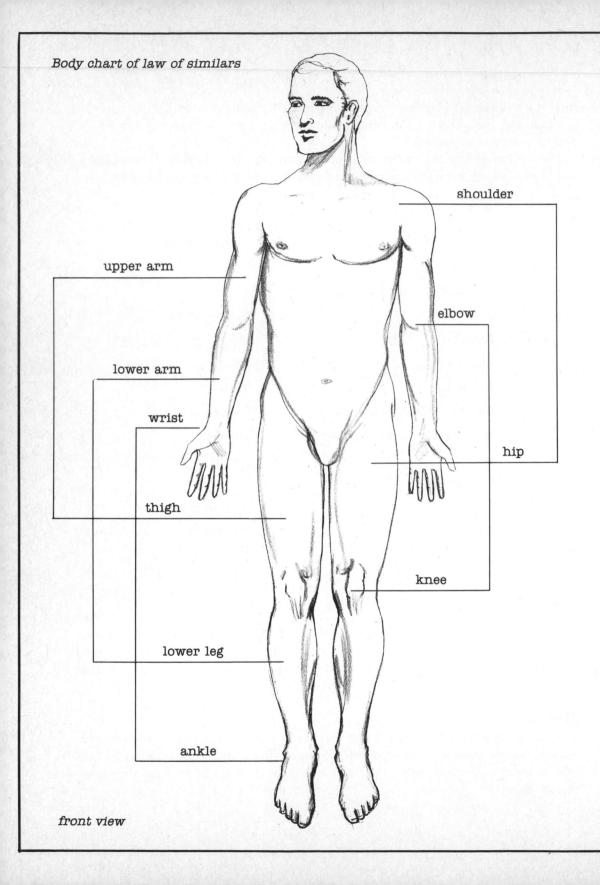

shoulder

upper arm

elbow

lower arm

wrist

hip

thigh

knee

lower leg

ankle

front view

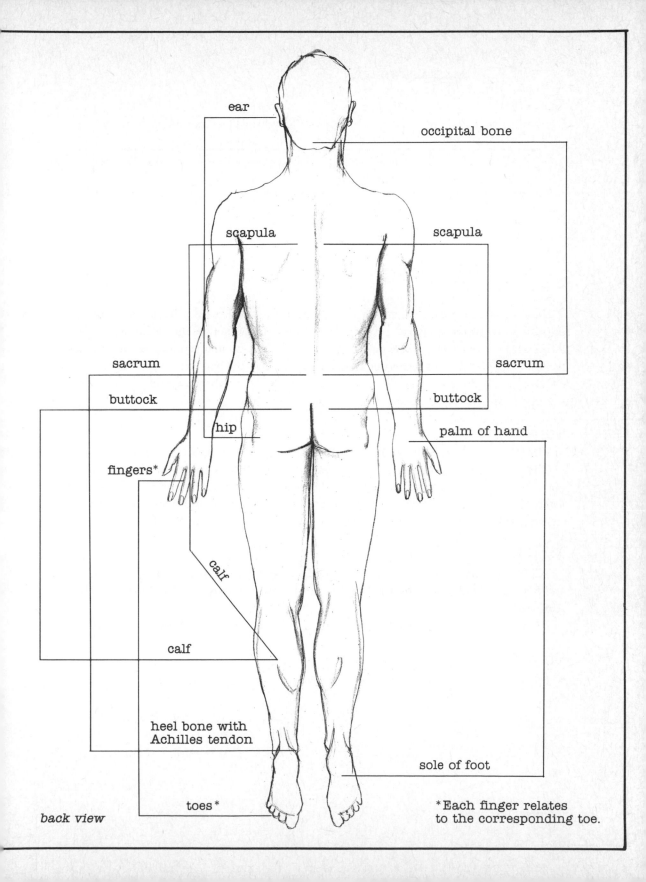

ear

occipital bone

scapula

scapula

sacrum

sacrum

buttock

buttock

hip

palm of hand

fingers*

calf

calf

heel bone with
Achilles tendon

sole of foot

toes*

back view

*Each finger relates
to the corresponding toe.

Step 3

If you choose, you may use gentle Circular Rhythmic Pressure on these points.

> **Remember:** *When doing a Law of Similars contact, it is important not to squeeze the body or to use heavy pressure.*

Muscle Squeeze

This technique is used when a muscle is underdeveloped, weak, flaccid, or tight. Its purpose is to bring strength and tone to the muscle. Although the technique is performed most easily on the legs, arms, and head, it can be done on any of the muscles listed in Chapter 2. This technique should be applied on the bare skin since it is not very effective when done through clothing. It is most effective when used on the buttocks, the upper and lower arms, and the upper and lower legs.

Step 1

Place one hand on either end of the muscle, near the surrounding joints.

This technique is always applied between two joints. For example, on the upper arm, place your hands firmly around the muscles that lie between the elbow and shoulder joint. Grasp the muscle firmly (but not so hard as to cause pain or discomfort) with your entire hand. Be careful not to dig into the muscle with your fingertips.

Step 2

With your hands around the muscle, firmly but gently press hands toward one another; then pull away so that the muscle is first manually contracted and then stretched.

If you are holding the muscle properly, friction and chafing will not take place.

Step 3

Repeat contraction and stretching ten times.

Vital Force Contact

This is the simplest and yet in many ways the most helpful of the nine techniques. It works totally on a vibrational or energy level as opposed to a structural level, and its purpose is to release the body's own self-healing energy wherever it is blocked in the body. Vital Force Contact is particularly recommended for injuries involving swelling, dislocations, fractures, or broken bones for which movement or manipulation of the joints is contraindicated. This technique is used when a person is so sensitive to touch that virtually any massage technique would create pain or discomfort.

For the development of your own sensitivity, it is good to apply this technique with your eyes closed. After about two or three minutes, you may begin to experience a sensation of heat or pulsation in your finger, hands, or arms. This means the energy blockage is opening up.

Step 1

With your index finger, use firm pressure to locate the point of blockage. You can ask your partner, "Where do you hurt?" or "Where do you feel tense?" Then instruct your partner to let you know when you touch a spot that is more sensitive than the rest of the area. If you have enough sensitivity in your fingers, you will probably feel a thickening or tightness of the muscle. If you have difficulty locating the precise point with your index finger, use your thumb and then switch to your index finger once you have located the blockage.

Step 2

Now rest your finger ever so lightly on the point. Then place your other hand on any joint of the body where it can rest comfortably. This second contact is made with the entire palm covering the joint and the fingers resting lightly on the body. Light pressure may be applied here, but it is not necessary. This hand serves as a grounding mechanism to help give form and direction to the energy as it circulates through the body. Maintain contact until you experience a sensation of heat in your index finger—about two to three minutes.

Remember: *This contact is a very subtle balancing tool. No benefit is gained from using pressure. Lightness of touch is really the key here.*

Muscle Kneading

This technique, which is similar to kneading dough, is used to stimulate the functions of the skin. It is especially good for skin that is very dry. In addition to the skin, it stimulates all the vital functions of the body part where it is applied: glands, nerves, and blood vessels as well as muscles and connective tissue. It is the only technique in our system for which oil is used on the skin of the person being massaged in order to reduce friction and chafing. After you apply a small film of oil on the skin (see section on oils at the end of this chapter), the kneading can begin.

Kneading is experienced by the body as an alternation between relaxation and compression. It helps to empty the blood and lymph vessels and to bring fresh fluid into these areas, thereby eliminating poisons and waste matter from the tissues and improving circulation. It is used routinely during warm-ups by dancers and athletes in order to reduce the possibility of injuries, cramps, and muscle spasms.

Step 1

After applying a small film of oil on the area to be worked on, grasp the muscle with a squeezing action of your hand. If the muscle is properly oiled, it will immediately begin to slip out of your hand.

Step 2

As the muscle slips from your hand, quickly grasp it with your other hand. The muscle will continue to slide from hand to hand as it is pressed, creating a rolling effect. Continue the kneading for about thirty seconds to one minute on most areas, but for about five minutes on the back.

Muscle kneading has many benefits. It is especially useful for firming weak muscles. Of all our bodywork techniques, this is probably the most structurally oriented. It is invaluable in paralysis and in all cases where there has been tissue degeneration. It can be applied easily anywhere on the body with the exception of the shin, bony joints, and the skull.

In working the muscles near a bone that had been fractured or near a sprain, Muscle Kneading is the technique to choose.

> **Caution:** *Avoid using this technique in any situation in which deep manipulation is contraindicated.*

Muscle Rock

This very gentle technique is used to release surface tension and superficial energy blocks in the body and to stimulate the sensory and motor nerves, thus readying the body for other techniques. Muscle Rock is excellent for removing both emotional and physical tension and consequently is a very good way to prepare the body for a complete massage session.

Step 1

Place the palm of your hand on the muscle to be rocked—where there is tension or discomfort. Use a very gentle touch with no pressure. Wrap your fingers around the muscle so that palm and fingers are touching the body. Rest your free hand on the joint above the area to be rocked. For example, if rocking the front thigh, rest the upper hand on the pelvic bone. If rocking the lower arm, rest the hand on the elbow joint. If rocking the buttocks, rest the upper hand on the back.

Step 2

With your hand resting firmly on the body part, slowly start to rock your palm back and forth in a firm, but nonforced movement. You can move your palm either horizontally or vertically. Rock for about two minutes.

> **Note:** *Make certain that your palm does not slide around (no lubricant is used). Do not grab, pinch, or press on the muscle.*

The Muscle Rock is a very soothing technique that seems to create a sense of tranquility between the giver and the receiver in much the same way that a mother's rocking has a soothing effect on both the mother and the baby.

> **Caution:** *Avoid using this technique in any situation where deep manipulation is contraindicated.*

General Rhythmic Pressure

There are two types of rhythmic pressure: general and circular. These techniques have a deeper effect than those previously described and are probably the most powerful of the nine techniques. In addition to pinpointing energy blockages, rhythmic pressure is also used to relieve deep-rooted muscle tension, structural problems, and restrictions in the range of motion. Rhythmic pressure is the technique to choose for muscle spasms and cramps and is one of the main techniques used to heal damaged tissue and reduce the formation of scar tissue after surgery or sprains.

General Rhythmic Pressure can be done very lightly or with firm pressure. We will indicate the amount of pressure by the terms "gentle," "firm," or "deep," but the amount of pressure used will depend on your or your partner's tolerance for pain. Whichever pressure is used, the approach is the same.

Step 1

Use your thumb to locate the tightness or knot in the muscle. This spot will probably be particularly sensitive.

Step 2

Using your body weight, press your thumb into the area *around* the discomfort. Hold the pressure for a couple of seconds and release; then apply again. Repeat as you move your thumb around the affected area in a clockwise direction. Do not slide the thumb across the skin. (In some situations it is preferable to use the heel of the hand. This is best determined case by case.)

When doing General Rhythmic Pressure it is often helpful to use a gentle Law of Similars reflex pressure on a corresponding body part. (See page 66).

> *Caution: Do not use this technique when the body temperature is higher or lower than normal. Never increase pressure suddenly—always apply it gradually, even when you are using deep pressure. And remember the guideline for applying pressure: never push forcefully with your finger. Instead, use your body weight to gradually increase the pressure.*

After General Rhythmic Pressure has been applied, Circular Rhythmic Pressure is the next technique to use.

Circular Rhythmic Pressure

Step 1

Slowly press your thumb down on the place where there is pain, spasm, or limited motion and rotate your thumb on this area in a clockwise motion. Do not slide it across the skin or lift it off the area. Revolve it slowly in one spot while manipulating the underlying muscle.

Step 2

As you move your thumb in a circular direction, increase the pressure. Some discomfort is expected, but *never* work so deeply as to cause extreme pain. As this circular pressure is applied, you may rhythmically increase and decrease the pressure in much the same way as in General Rhythmic Pressure.

Gradually the spasm or knot will begin to loosen up and disappear. Either you will feel this happening with your thumb or the person receiving the massage will experience less discomfort, or both.

Also, you may experience a sensation of heat or pulsation in your thumb. Although it is possible that you are feeling your own pulse beat, if the pulse increases or decreases, you are most likely feeling the opening up of the blockage. You should continue with the revolving, circular motion until the discomfort subsides.

> **Note:** *The contraindications for Circular Rhythmic Pressure are the same as those for General Rhythmic Pressure.*

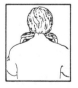

Pull and Stretch

This is a fairly simple technique applied to the legs. While your partner is lying on his or her back, grasp one of your partner's feet in each hand and, holding them firmly, slowly and steadily lean all of your body weight backward. This should give a good stretch to your partner's hip and lower back muscles.

> **Caution:** *Avoid using this technique on people suffering from bone disorders or those who have had recent hip, knee, or ankle injuries.*

In addition to the nine techniques we have outlined, there are a few more things you should know before giving a massage.

Touch

Before you massage yourself or someone else, you must first develop a sensitive touch. A keen sense of touch will enable you to locate blockages as well as determine when a technique is achieving the desired results. Through your sense of touch you can communicate with the body and let the body speak for itself. Your fingers will be able to pick up the messages that the body is sending about its condition.

A good way to develop a sensitive touch is to work on yourself or a partner with your eyes closed. After using firm pressure with your finger to locate a blockage, rest your finger lightly on the spot. A blockage is indicated when you feel tightness in the muscle or when a spot is particularly sensitive to touch. Within two or three minutes you should feel a warm sensation or a strong pulse beat. This indicates that the blockage is loosening.

The pressure that you use in massage can be either light and gentle or heavy and deep. The amount of pressure you use and the effect it has will differ, depending on the individual, the body part, the particular problem, and the specific technique. There are, however, some general rules that apply to the use of pressure:

○ All initial body contacts should be made with a firm pressure.
○ Light, quick pressure tends to have a tonifying (stimulating) effect on the body. Deep, sustained pressure usually has a sedative (calming) or even at times a numbing effect.
○ Never apply pressure on a bony prominence, such as the ankle, wrist, knee, or collarbone, since this will restrict circulation and can also injure a nerve.
○ Never push forcefully with your finger. Instead, use your body weight to increase pressure gradually. In other words, lean your body into the pressure rather than simply bearing down or pressing with your finger. This concept is crucial to our techniques, and with experience you will be able to make the distinction.

○ Never apply direct pressure on a painful point. Instead, apply gradually increasing pressure on the surrounding area rather than on the painful area itself. This will increase circulation and balance energy. If deep pressure is placed directly on a painful area, your partner will probably become more tense and the effectiveness of the technique you are using will be diminished.

Many massage and bodywork techniques are based on the premise that the heavier the pressure, the more effective it will be. This notion is especially widespread among practitioners of structure-based systems that attempt to affect the structure and functions of bones, connective tissues, and muscles, for example in techniques such as reflexology and Rolfing.

Though there certainly are times when strong pressure may bring very positive results, our experience has taught us that a skillfully placed, sensitive hand can produce satisfactory results with a minimum of pressure. Too much pressure can be dangerous, causing damage to nerves or bones, and even paralysis.

On the other hand, some practitioners believe that if enough pressure is applied, the body will always react with pain or sensitivity. Our experience indicates, however, that when the body is healthy, there will be little or no pain, even when heavy pressure is applied.

Although many people are comfortable with and may even prefer a heavy approach, others react with intense pain to even a seemingly light touch. Be sensitive. Ask your partner for feedback. Watch for facial expressions and body tensions that show discomfort.

Dialogue is most important to determine the appropriate pressure. Many people erroneously believe that the greater the pain, the greater the benefit, and they will attempt to be stoic "for their own good." Make certain that your partner clearly understands that he or she should tell you if the pain becomes sharp or intense. As you increase the pressure ask your partner, "How does this feel?" or "Does this hurt?"

Breathing and Relaxation

Before doing bodywork on yourself or someone else, you should be as relaxed as possible, both physically and emotionally. Your entire body, but especially your hands, should feel light and loose before you touch yourself or your partner.

As a loosening exercise, try the following:

1. Slowly shake your hands until you feel free of tension.

2. Take three very slow, deep breaths—breathing in for the count of four, holding for the count of six, and exhaling for the count of eight.

Once you feel thoroughly relaxed and your hands hang limp from your wrists, you may begin.

After you begin, it is important to maintain a steady breathing rhythm, since your energy and your relaxation are directly affected by your breathing pattern. Try to breathe in rhythm with your partner. This makes the balancing effect more profound and creates a strong connection between the two of you. You might try having your partner breathe along with you during the loosening exercise. Another technique for developing rhythmic harmony is to place your hand on your partner's abdomen to pick up his or her breathing pattern.

There are other ways to free yourself of tension before doing a massage, such as short meditation or listening to soothing music. The important thing is that your hands and body are warm and free—never cold, tight, or tense.

Precautions: When Not to Massage

When doing any form of bodywork or body manipulation, it is important to recognize that certain techniques are contraindicated for certain medical conditions. A full description of possible anatomical and physiological precautionary factors go beyond the scope of this book. However, the following is a list of physical conditions that generally require caution. If you have any of these problems, or any others that you think could create difficulties, check with your physician before receiving a massage that involves deep pressure or manipulation.

○ recently torn tendons, ligaments, or muscles
○ osteoporosis
○ osteoarthritis where a danger of fracturing exists
○ osteoarthritis where active inflammation exists (signaled by heat, redness, and soreness)
○ skin, muscle, and bone diseases, including active infections under the skin
○ unhealed bone fractures
○ hypertension
○ cancerous tumor

- ○ heart condition
- ○ diabetes
- ○ fever
- ○ frostbite
- ○ acute inflammation (bodywork may be applied to uninflamed parts)
- ○ any form of skin disease *except* thickened skin left by chronic eczema.
- ○ tubercular joints
- ○ aneurisms (dilation of an artery)
- ○ thrombosis (an obstruction in a blood vessel, caused by blood clotting)
- ○ acute inflammation of the kidneys

With diabetics, use only light techniques, such as gentle Vital Force Contact, a light Muscle Rock, or light General Rhythmic Pressure. Deep work on the extremities can place dangerous stresses on arteries and veins. Gentle Muscle Kneading, however, will improve muscle tone and increase circulation.

When working on pregnant women, techniques should always be applied gently, never deeply or heavily. Your partner should always lie on her back or side, never on her stomach.

If a person has specific medical problems that prevent or restrict active exercise, use our passive exercises described in Chapter 8. These simple stretching movements develop and energize the muscles without exhausting them, stimulate the circulatory system without placing unnecessary stress on the heart, and feed the muscles as well as vital energy centers without exhausting or taxing the nervous system.

Clothing

If you find it necessary to work on someone who is wearing heavy clothing, do so, but keep in mind that this will definitely interfere with your sense of touch and may prevent your partner from being as relaxed as possible. Suitable apparel for the person who is being massaged is a pair of gym trunks for men and a bikini swimsuit for women.

Although massage can be performed through clothing, we have found that its effectiveness is greatly diminished, particularly when the clothing is made from synthetic fibers. We recommend that both you and your partner wear a natural fiber such as cotton, wool, silk, or linen.

Creams and Oils

Creams and oils are used for their specific healing properties and/or to eliminate friction in massage. There are several oils that may be used. A simple vegetable oil, like safflower or sesame oil, or pure olive oil, can be used to reduce friction. However, many of these oils may stain clothing or sheets. This is not a problem, however, with most of the aromatic or essential plant oils, such as wintergreen or oil of clove, since they evaporate fairly quickly, but because they evaporate quickly they cannot be used alone for massage and must be mixed with a vegetable oil. Both essential and aromatic oils will also give you greater flexibility and can be used in your bath as well as in inhalers and vaporizers.

Many bodywork practitioners use organic coconut oil. Though it is solid in the jar, it quickly melts when applied to the body. Not only is it easy to work with, but it is odorless, inexpensive, will not stain clothing or sheets, and is the least allergenic oil. Also worth considering are many of the premixed oils available in health-food stores.

Do not pour oil directly on the body from the jar. First rub it on your hands until it is warm and then rub it over your partner's body. By touching the oil first, the warmth of your hands will bring it close to normal body temperature.

Remember: *Ask your partner if he or she is allergic to any oils.*

The Working Area Placing a sheet over a rug will give you a good working area on the floor. For a good session, the work surface should not be too hard nor too soft. Most mattresses are too soft, and beds are not usually a good choice for a massage surface because they do not support. Some people may find it uncomfortable to work on the floor. In such situations you may wish to place a thick pad or quilt on a long table. The person giving the massage may proceed with the session in either a standing or sitting position. Many massage therapists use professional massage tables and excellent ones can be built or purchased.

These massage techniques, if used regularly and sensitively—together with good nutrition and proper exercise—can help you become healthier and feel more relaxed and alive. In the following chapters we will explain how the techniques we have described can be used in doing a full massage session for a partner or on yourself to help reduce aches and pains and provide an increased sense of well-being.

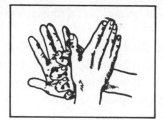

CHAPTER 4

DOING A FULL MASSAGE SESSION

Once the nine basic techniques have been learned, you may want to do a full massage session that is not directed to any specific problem. You must start by being in touch with your partners mood and flow of vital energy. You will learn how much pressure to give and how much to work a particular body part as you practice, but until you become more experienced, it is best to begin each movement slowly and gradually, constantly watching your partner's face and general reactions. You may also ask along the way if you are applying too much, or even too little, pressure.

Techniques such as General Rhythmic Pressure are geared to relax and prepare the muscles for deeper pressure. Vital Force Contact and Law of Similars are deeper techniques that effect a more drastic change. The Muscle Rock is also a preparatory movement that helps ready the body for deeper massage. If you simply want to give a good massage to make your partner feel better, a gentle Muscle Rock and Rhythmic Pressure will relax the muscles and remove knots of tension that may cause blockages to your partner's overall energy flow.

When the body is overstimulated or the blood pressure is higher than normal, the body needs to relax. The general method is to use long and deep strokes. The penetration should gradually be deepened and the amount of time for each movement should be longer. The opposite applies if the body is tired or lacks energy. It needs to be stimulated. In this case, it is best to work shallowly and quickly to effect a tonifying change on the entire system. By working in short and quick movements, you will activate the body's vital force and strengthen this energy flow.

However, keep in mind also that there may be times when you may use short, quick movements on one part of the body and use long deep techniques on another part of the body, all in the same session.

We have found that the time for each movement can vary, but the length of each session is usually at least one hour, but not longer than an hour and a half. If you are addressing a particular part of the body, such as the head to relieve a headache, you could massage for about fifteen or twenty minutes just that part alone. After you have done several full massage sessions as outlined in this chapter, you will start to know how long each technique should take and be able to adjust the times for different body parts.

An important general rule is to never apply pressure in one spot for longer than five minutes at any one time. Release the pressure and start it again. After too long a period of applying pressure, the body can start to get numb, because the circulation is cut off.

Many people will wait until a crisis occurs before they pay attention to the care of the body, but often injuries and illnesses can be prevented by keeping the body fit and healthy. Staying limber, but firm, and maintaining a strong respiratory system enables us to resist the wear and tear that is associated with the stress and overwork most of us experience. Our full body massage procedures focus on preventing problems in the body or, at least, correcting them before they become severe and cause pain or difficulty in movement. Unlike acupressure or polarity, which are energy-based systems, and chiropractic, Rolfing, and Swedish massage, which are primarily structure-based methods, our system emphasizes strengthening the body's own self-healing energy flow, tonifying the muscles, and effecting the body's chemical balance.

Head

Start with Vital Force Contact. This is a very powerful technique for relaxing the entire system and creating a bond of trust and sharing between you and your partner. It will bring both of you in touch with your emotional centers, break down emotional armor, and begin a reciprocal flow of vital life energy between you.

1. Have your partner lie on her back with legs flat and arms straight at sides.

2. While you are standing at the end of the table near your partner's head, gently cradle her head in the palms of your hands, with your fingers gently resting on the base of the skull. Do not apply any pressure. Tell your partner, "Just let your head relax totally in my hands." The head should rest in your hands as if on a pillow.

3. Tell your partner to place her hands on her abdomen and breathe deeply and rhythmically into abdominal area three times, inhaling to the count of nine and exhaling to the count of three. Hold this position for about three minutes.

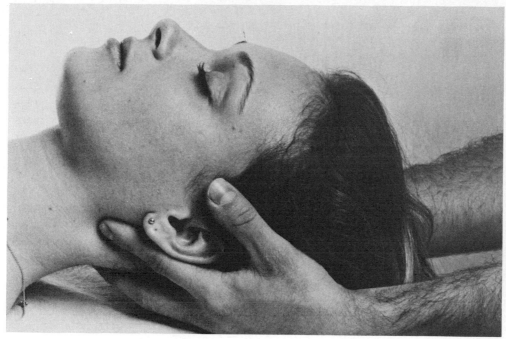

Head cradle

4. Now tell your partner to visualize the oxygen bringing relaxation into the body and taking tension out: "Feel your muscles relaxing."

5. Next, as you begin to feel warmth in your hands, coordinate your breathing with your partner's. Close your eyes and hold this position for two to three minutes. Now remove your hands very slowly. If your partner indicates in any way that she would like to hold this position for a while longer, return your hands. It can be disquieting to your partner if you remove your hands prematurely, since this contact produces a sensation of having the entire body cradled and is extremely comforting.

Back

Next, have your partner turn over on her stomach. Stand at the side of the table. Place a small pillow (like a baby's pillow) or a folded towel under your partner's head so that

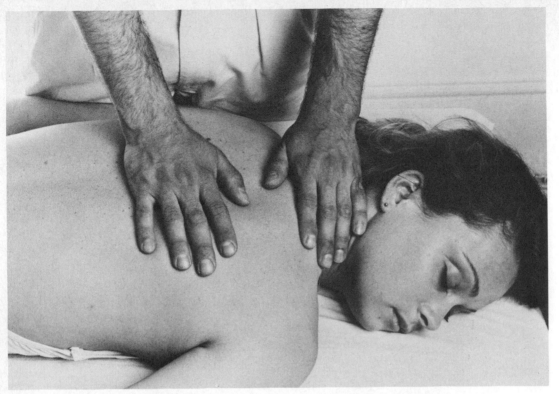

Muscle Rock: Where to place hands on spine

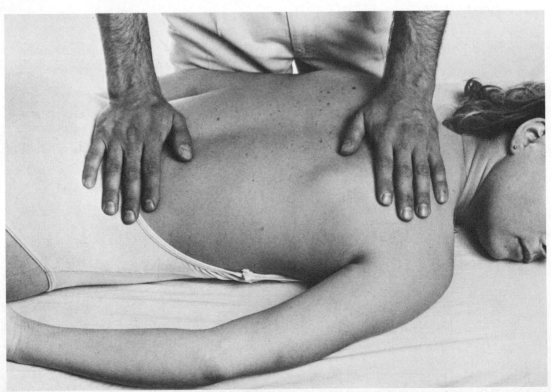

Muscle Rock: Hands moving down spine

the neck and head are even with the shoulders; otherwise there will be strain in the neck.

Begin with a Muscle Rock down each side of the spine. This technique stimulates circulation and provides a feeling of general well-being to the whole body. As you gain experience you will be able to use this technique to notice problem areas in other parts of the body because the stable hand will feel heat or pulsation whenever the moving hand makes contact with a reflex point for an area of imbalance.

1. Place both your hands over your partner's spine, your upper hand (which is the stable hand) at the base of the neck and the lower hand (which is the moving hand) next to it. Your hands should be lightly curved, with the fingertips barely resting on your partner's back. Now rock nine times, using gentle pressure with the palms. *Be careful not to press on the spine.*

2. Now move the bottom hand about four inches down the back, keeping the upper hand in place, and rock.

3. You should keep moving the lower hand down the back in this way about four inches each time, until you reach the end of your partner's spine.

4. Now move your hands back to the starting position, but with your palms resting on the other side of the spine, about two inches away, and repeat the process.

Next apply General Rhythmic Pressure to the spine with your palms.

1. Place your hands on your partner's back with the palms resting in the spinal groove (see Fig. 24). The top hand should be at the base of the neck with the bottom hand next to it, as in the Muscle Rock.

2. Make sure to keep the upper hand in place and move the lower hand slowly down the back (taking care to stay in the spinal groove), applying firm General Rhythmic Pressure down to the end of the spine. Apply pressure six times in each spot, moving the hand about four inches at a time.

3. Move the hands to the other side of the spine, with the palms in the spinal groove, and, starting at the top, repeat the process. Now apply Circular Rhythmic Pressure with the thumbs on both sides of the spine.

1. Starting at the base of the neck, place one hand on each side of the spine with the thumbs in the spinal groove. Moving down the spine with both hands, about one inch at a time, apply gentle Circular Rhythmic Pressure all the way to the end of the spine.

Finish working on the back with Muscle Kneading.

1. Starting just below the bottom tip of the shoulder blade (scapula), grasp the muscle between the thumb and the index finger of one hand, close to the shoulder blade. Lift and squeeze as firmly as possible. As the flesh slips away, grasp it with the other hand. Repeat this movement, alternating hands, and work down to the end of the spine. It may be a little difficult to do this on the lower back, but give it a try.

2. Now work your way back up to the shoulder blade.

3. Repeat process on the other side of back.

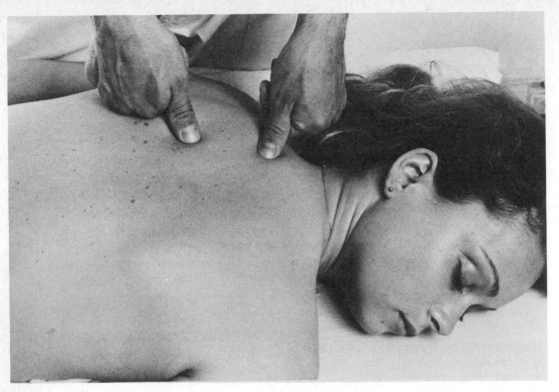

Circular Rhythmic Pressure: Where to place thumbs on spine

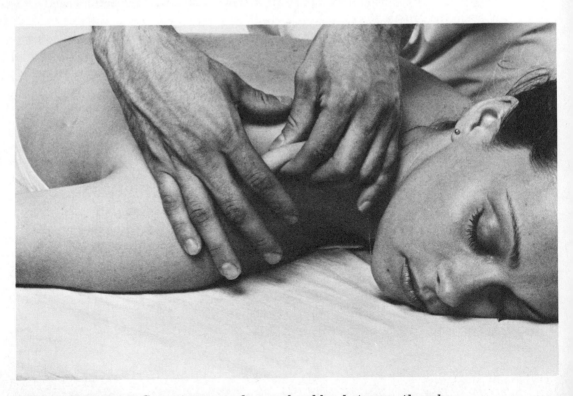

Muscle Kneading: Grasping muscle on shoulder between thumbs and index fingers

Buttocks

The buttocks are a very sensitive area that many people associate with sensuous feelings. They are a storage area for fear, anger, and sexual energy. Some people will find work on this area very pleasant, others might resist having the buttocks touched at all. However, most people like it, and work on the buttocks can be pleasurable, as well as therapeutic—tonifying the buttocks muscles and relieving tensions in the thighs and lower back.

Begin with the Muscle Squeeze. Place hands on each side of the buttocks. Squeeze the buttocks together between the hands and hold for the count of five. Repeat three times.

Muscle Squeeze on buttocks

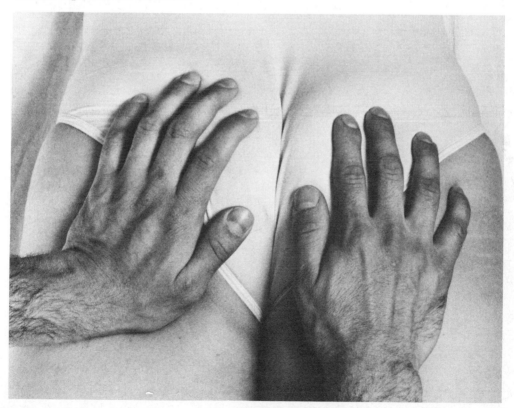

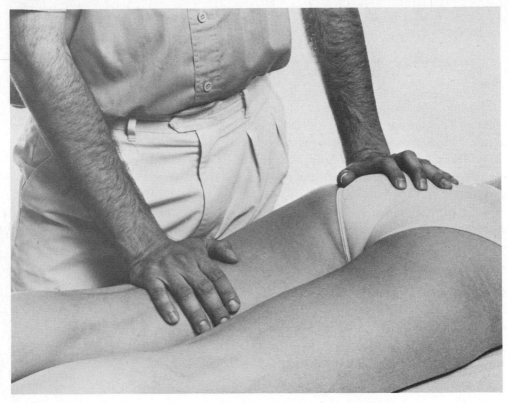

Law of Similars, buttocks to calf: Placement of hands

Next apply General Rhythmic Pressure. Place both hands at the top of one buttock. Using both thumbs at once, apply Rhythmic Pressure over the entire buttock for two to three minutes. Repeat on other buttock. On each buttock, start with gentle pressure and gradually increase to firm pressure.

Finish the buttocks by using the Law of Similars—buttocks to calf.

1. With one hand press firmly into the calf with your thumb until you find a sensitive spot. Now place your middle finger of the same hand on that point and hold it.

2. With the thumb of your other hand, locate a sensitive point in the buttock on the same side of the body. Once you find a sensitive spot, replace your thumb with your index finger.

3. In general, hold the contacts until you feel heat or pulsation.

4. Repeat the process on other side of the body. This technique creates an equilibrium in the lower back and legs.

Legs

Begin with a Muscle Rock to the back of the legs.

1. Place one hand just below the buttocks. Place the other hand (the lower, moving one) directly on the bend of the knee. Now rock your hands gently nine times.

2. Moving the lower hand about three inches at a time, proceed down to the ankle, rocking nine times every three inches.

3. Repeat for the other leg.

Next apply Muscle Kneading to the back of the legs.

Muscle Rock, back of leg: Where to place hands

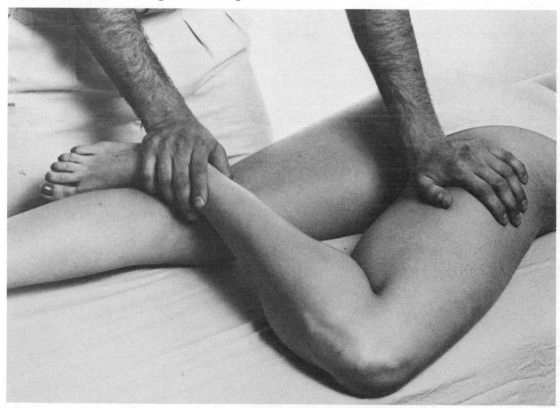

1. Place both hands on back of your partner's thigh, immediately below the buttocks. Starting with the lower hand, firmly grasp a portion of the thigh between the thumb and fingers and knead to the knee. Then knead the calf to the ankle. Imagine you are kneading dough.

2. Repeat for the other leg. *Do not knead at knee or ankle.*

Now apply General Rhythmic Pressure to the back of the legs.

1. Place your hands on your partner's thigh, just below the buttocks. Keep the upper hand stable.

2. With the other, moving hand, apply General Rhythmic Pressure with palm down to the knee. Apply the pressure by leaning your body weight gently into your hand. *Do not apply Rhythmic Pressure behind knee.*

When doing this, apply Rhythmic Pressure from just below knee to the heel of the foot. *Do not apply Rhythmic Pressure to ankle.*

The Range of Motion for the front of the legs is the back knee bend.

1. Move to the foot of the massage table.

Range of Motion: Back knee bend

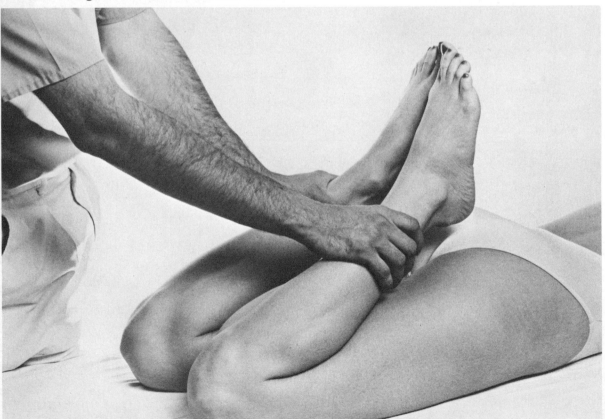

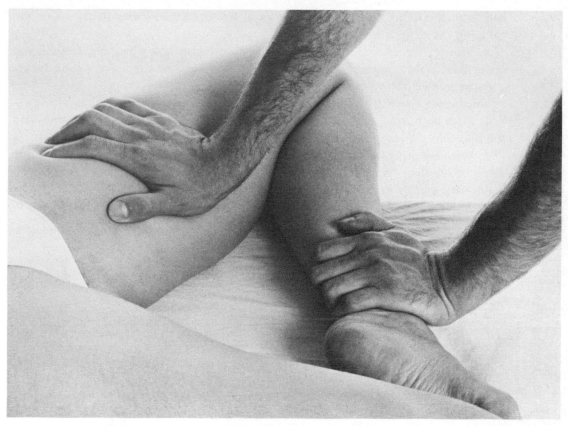

Muscle Rock, side of leg: Hand placement and position

2. Place the palm of one hand on the top of each of your partner's feet.

3. Holding the feet firmly, bend both your partner's legs at the knee and press feet toward buttocks. Stop when you feel resistance.

Remember: Never force a body part beyond its comfortable range of motion. Bending both legs at the same time will help you determine which leg is tighter and more in need of attention. You can then perform more Range of Motion on this leg in order to develop a balance between the two. The goal is eventually to get both heels to be able to lie against the buttocks.

Continue with a Muscle Rock to the outside of the legs.

1. Move to the side of the table.

2. Cross one of your partner's ankles over the knee of her other leg.

3. Place one hand on the outside of the leg just below the buttocks. Put the other

hand directly in the bend of the straight knee. Now rock your hands gently nine times, applying the motion with your palms.

4. Moving the second, lower hand about three inches at a time, and keeping your upper hand stable, proceed down to the ankle, rocking nine times every three inches.

5. Repeat for the other leg.

Next apply General Rhythmic Pressure to the outside of the legs.

1. Place both hands on outside of the thigh just below the buttocks. Keep one hand, the upper one, stable.

2. With the other (moving) hand, apply Rhythmic Pressure with your palm, moving down to the knee. Apply the pressure by leaning your body weight gently into your hand. *Do not apply Rhythmic Pressure to knee.*

3. Apply Rhythmic Pressure from just below the knee to the heel of the foot. *Do not apply Rhythmic Pressure to ankle.*

Law of Similars, sacrum to heel: Where to place hands

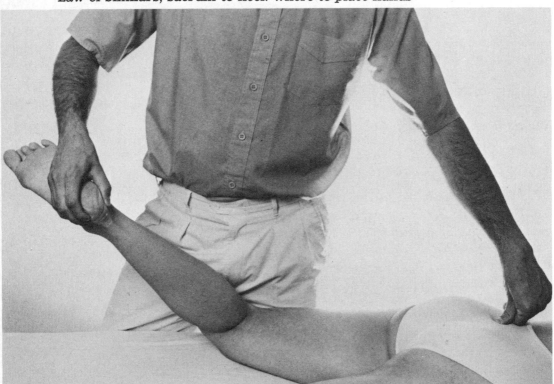

Apply the Law of Similars—sacrum to heel.

1. With the thumb of one hand locate a sensitive point on the heel. Once you have found a sensitive spot, replace your thumb with your middle finger.

2. Now locate your partner's sacrum, by locating the top of the pelvic (hip) bone. With your finger, draw an imaginary horizontal line to the spine. This is the point. Now place the thumb of your other hand on this spot.

3. Hold the contacts until you feel heat or pulsation.

4. Repeat the process on the other leg.

Continue with Law of Similars—buttock to shoulder blade (scapula).

1. With the thumb of one hand locate a sensitive point on the buttocks. Now replace your thumb with your middle finger.

2. With the thumb of your upper hand, locate a sensitive point near the center of the shoulder blade. Now replace your thumb with your index finger.

Law of Similars, buttocks to shoulder blade: Where to place hands

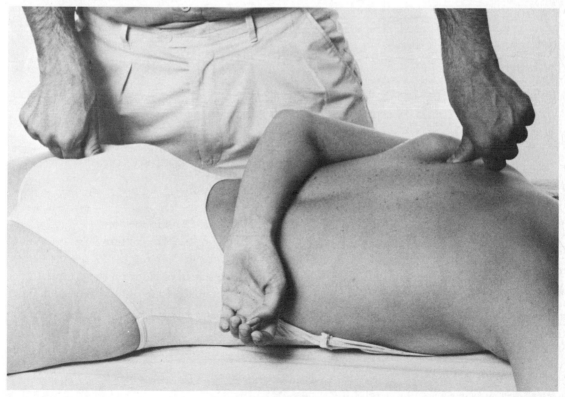

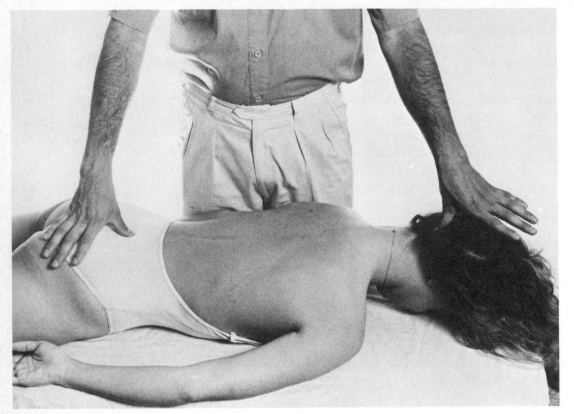

Law of Similars, sacrum to occipital bone: Where to place hands

3. Hold the contacts until you feel heat or pulsation.

4. Repeat process on other side of body.

Finish the legs with the Law of Similars—sacrum to occipital bone.

1. With the thumb of one hand, locate the sacrum (see Law of Similars—sacrum to heel, above) and then replace your thumb with your middle finger.

2. With the thumb of your other hand, locate a sensitive point on the occipital bone (the bony ridge where the spine joins the skull). Replace your thumb with your index finger.

3. Hold the contacts until you feel heat or pulsation.

Now ask your partner to turn over on her back.

Abdomen

Begin with a Muscle Rock. This is a very pleasant and soothing technique that owners of cats and dogs use on their pets all the time. Every time your pet turns over on her back and looks at you longingly, she's asking for a Muscle Rock. Mothers also do this to their babies to help put them to sleep.

1. Place your upper hand on your partner's forehead. Place your bottom hand on your partner's abdomen.

2. With the slightest pressure on the palm of your hand, gently rock the abdomen from side to side. Do this for about thirty seconds.

In addition to being very soothing, this technique is useful for releasing trapped gas and balancing abdominal organs.

Where to place hands on abdomen for Muscle Rock

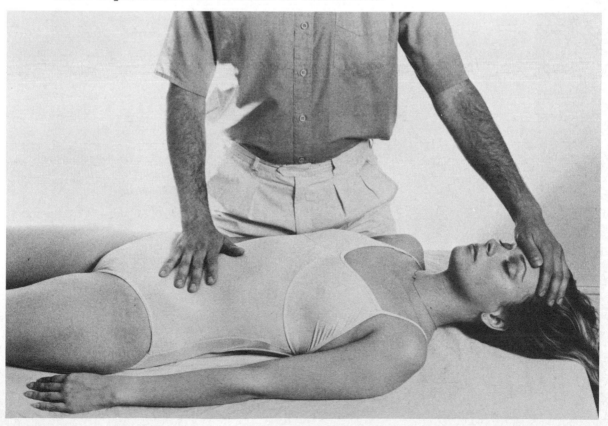

Ankles, Feet and Toes

Start by using Range of Motion for the ankles.

1. Holding your partner's leg just above the ankle with one hand, clasp his toes in your other hand and firmly rotate them six times clockwise and six times counter-clockwise.

2. Repeat for the other foot.

Repeat Range of Motion for the toes.

1. Stabilize your partner's foot by clasping the foot with your palm under the sole.

2. Rotate one toe at a time, three times clockwise and three times counterclockwise.

Range of Motion: How to rotate ankle
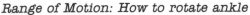

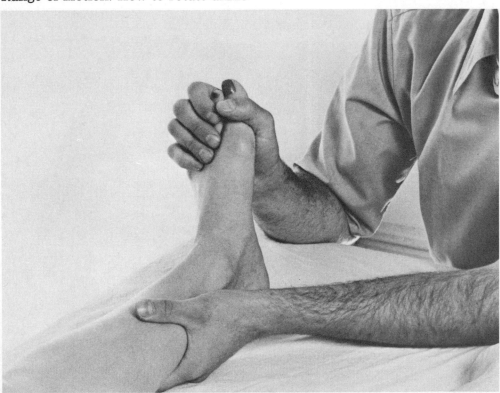

3. Repeat for the other foot.

Next apply a Muscle Squeeze to each foot.

1. Place your hand under the sole of your partner's foot at the metatarsal arch, and firmly squeeze the foot.

2. Hold for the count of five. Repeat three times.

3. Repeat for the other foot.

Apply Circular Rhythmic Pressure to the entire foot.

1. Hold your partner's foot with one hand. With the thumb of the other hand, perform Circular Rhythmic Pressure over the top and sole of the foot and the toes. Spend about twice as much time on the sole, since the bottom of the foot is the storehouse for reflex points throughout the body.

2. Repeat for the other foot.

Legs

Begin with a Pull and Stretch of the legs.

1. While standing at the foot of the table, firmly grasp one of your partner's feet in each of your hands.

2. Slowly lean your body backward, pulling the legs as you go and balancing yourself with your partner's body.

3. When you reach the point of resistance, hold for thirty seconds and then relax.

4. Repeat three times. (See Fig. page 63).

Next perform a Muscle Rock to the front of the legs.

1. Move to the side of the table.

2. Place one hand at the very top of the thigh. Put the other hand directly on the knee. Now rock your hands gently nine times.

3. Moving the lower hand about three inches at a time, proceed down to the ankle, rocking nine times every three inches.

4. Repeat for the other leg.

Use Muscle Kneading on the front of the legs.

1. Place both hands on top of the thigh. With one hand, grasp a portion of the thigh between the thumb and four fingers and knead to the knee. Imagine you are kneading dough.

2. Repeat for the other leg. *Do not knead knee, shin or ankle.*

Apply General Rhythmic Pressure to the inside of the legs.

1. Cross your partner's ankle over the knee of his other foot.

2. Now place both your hands on the inside top of his thigh. Keep one hand stable.

3. With the lower, moving hand, apply Rhythmic Pressure with the palm, down to the knee. Apply the pressure by leaning your body weight gently into your hand. *Do not apply Rhythmic Pressure on the knee.*

4. Apply Rhythmic Pressure to the calf and the heel. *Do not apply Rhythmic Pressure to the ankle.*

5. Now, using your thumbs, apply Rhythmic Pressure to the inside of the thigh and calf.

6. Repeat for the other leg.

The Range of Motion for the back of the legs is the front knee bend.

1. Move to the end of the table.

2. Put your hands under both of your partner's knees and bend knees toward partner's chest. Stop when you feel resistance. This technique determines the tightness in the hamstrings (back thigh tendons).

As with the back knee bend, bending both legs at the same time will help you determine which leg is tighter and more in need of attention. You can then do more Range of Motion with the tighter leg in order to develop a balance between the two. The goal is to get both knees to lie flat against the chest.

Range of Motion, front knee bend

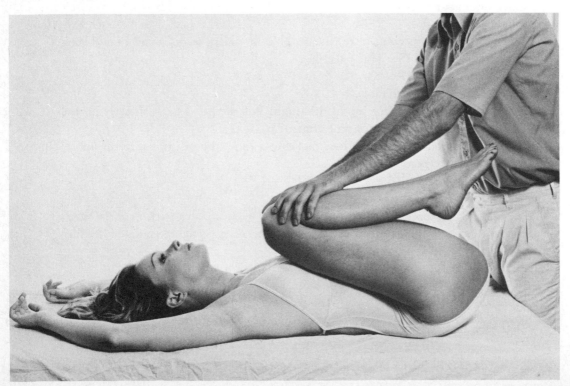

Chest

Apply Circular Rhythmic Pressure.

1. Return to the side of the table.

2. Place your hands on the chest. Apply gentle Circular Rhythmic Pressure. Be careful not to apply too much pressure because there are several delicate bones in the chest area.

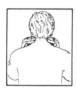

Shoulder and Upper Arms

Begin with the Law of Similars—upper arm to thigh.

Law of Similars, upper arm to thigh: Where to place hands

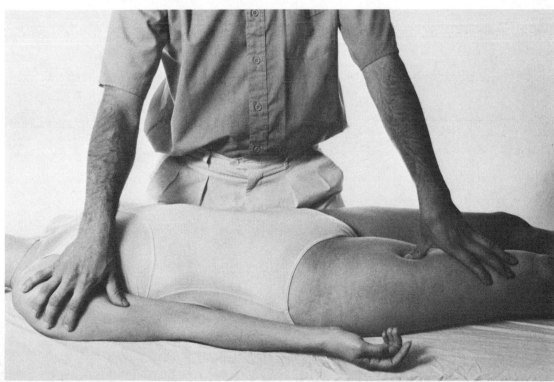

1. With the thumb of one hand, locate a sensitive point on the upper arm; replace your thumb with your index finger.

2. With the thumb of your other hand, locate a sensitive point on the thigh, then replace thumb with middle finger.

3. Hold the contacts until you feel heat or pulsation.

4. Repeat process on the other side.

Now apply the Range of Motion to each shoulder.

1. With one hand stabilizing the shoulder, clasp your partner's fingers with your other hand.

2. Now using your lower hand, rotate the entire arm, six times clockwise and six times counterclockwise.

3. Repeat for the other side.

Elbows and Wrists

Begin with Range of Motion.

1. With your upper hand holding the middle of your partner's upper arm, grasp her wrist and rotate the elbow six times clockwise and six times counterclockwise.

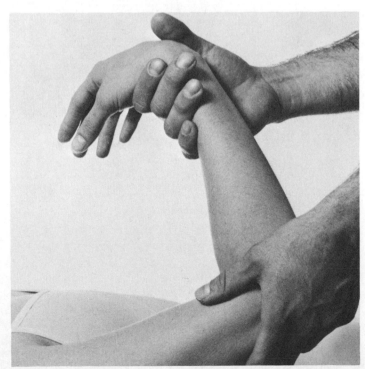

Range of Motion:
How to rotate elbow

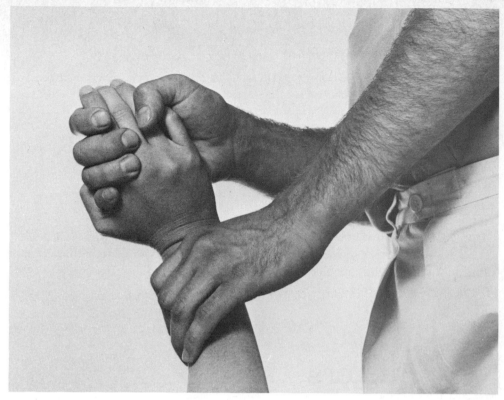

Range of Motion: How to rotate wrist

Range of Motion: How to rotate fingers

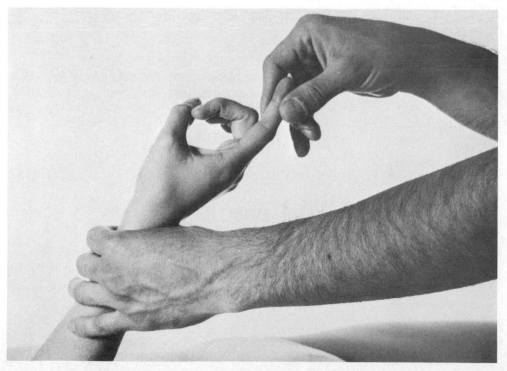

2. Supporting the middle of his forearm with one hand, and clasping his fingers with your other hand, rotate the wrist six times clockwise and six times counterclockwise.

3. Repeat for the other side.

Hands

Apply Circular Rhythmic Pressure.

1. Hold your partner's hand in both of yours, and with both of your thumbs apply Circular Rhythmic Pressure over the entire palm of the hand and the fingers.

2. Repeat for the other hand.

Fingers

Begin with Range of Motion on each finger.

1. Isolate the finger you are working on by clasping the other fingers in your hand.

2. Use the other hand to rotate each finger individually, three times clockwise and three times counterclockwise.

3. Repeat for the other hand.

Apply Muscle Kneading to each finger.

1. Rest your partner's elbow on the table or the palm of your free hand.

2. Working from thumb to the little finger, knead your partner's fingers by rubbing your thumb and index finger slowly and firmly over his. Work from the base of each finger to the tip.

3. Repeat on the other hand.

Head and Neck

Begin with Range of Motion for head and neck.

1. Stand behind your partner's head. Form the letter X with your arms. Place the center of the X under your partner's head and place your hands on the tops of your partner's shoulders.

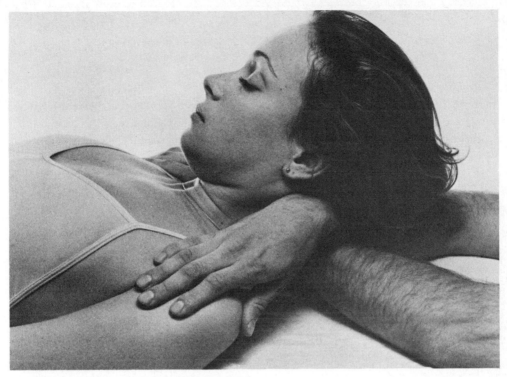

Range of Motion: How to rotate neck

2. Now gently and rhythmically use your body to raise your arms to the left, thereby lifting your partner's head. Slowly return to center.

3. Lift your partners head to the right. Return to center. Now lift forward. Hold each position for the count of six.

This is a very powerful movement, which stretches the cervical and thoracic vertebrae and increases circulation to the head. It creates a flowing sense of harmony between the giver and the receiver.

Continue with Range of Motion by circling the head.

1. Place one hand on each side of your partner's head with your palms lightly cupping his·or her eyes.

2. Now gently turn the head to the right and hold for the count of six; return to center; then slowly turn to the left and hold for the count of six. Return.

Next apply Circular Rhythmic Pressure to the neck.

1. Slowly and gently apply Circular Rhythmic Pressure to the sides of the neck. When you find a tight area, slowly increase the pressure.

> ***Caution:*** *do not press too firmly on the blood vessels in the neck. If your partner indicates that you are working with too firm a touch, lighten the pressure.*

Now use Muscle Kneading on each ear.

Grasp the earlobe between the thumb and index finger. Slowly rub the earlobe. Then move from the lobe to cover the entire outer edge of the ear. This produces an exhilarating feeling and may be done with oil, which will heighten the experience.

Finally, apply General Rhythmic Pressure to the eyes.

Briskly rub the palms of your hands together to create heat and increase circulation. Now place your hands over your partner's eyes and very gently apply pressure with the palms. Hold for about thirty seconds.

General Rhythmic Pressure to the eyes

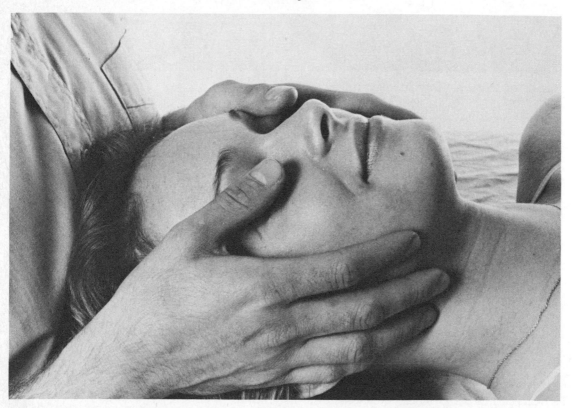

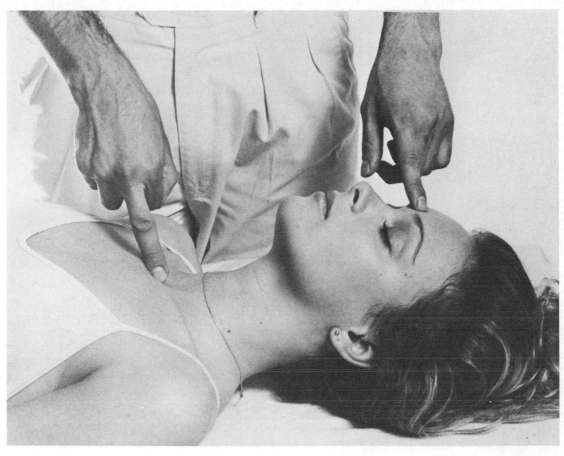

Three-point Vital Force Contact: Third eye to crest of sternum

Now it's time to bring your bodywork session full circle. Repeat the Head Cradle. Then bring it all together using a three-point Vital Force Contact.

1. Place your one index finger in the center of the forehead, between the eyebrows (third eye). Place the other index finger at the crest of the sternum, where the collar bones meet. Hold for at least a minute.

2. Move the finger from the forehead and place it gently over the navel. Keep the other finger on the sternum, and hold for a minute.

3. Move the finger over the sternum back to the third eye. Hold it there for a minute.

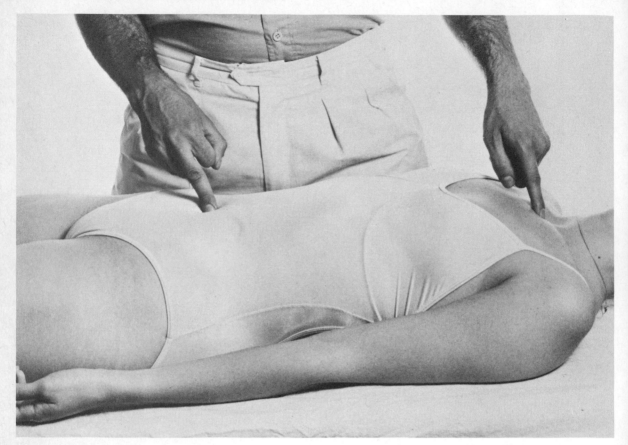

Crest of Sternum to navel

We have found that, after finishing, if you lightly move your hands across your partner's body in a sort of sweeping motion away from the head toward the feet and make a positive statement, such as "have good health," and take a deep breath, this will ground you and your partner, and complete a pleasant experience.

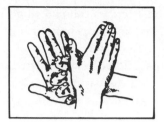

CHAPTER 5

DO IT YOURSELF

Most systems of massage require someone to give the massage and someone to receive it. There are a number of moves and techniques in our system that do not require two people, so we have devised a massage series that is useful for general massage and for specific problems that can be done without anyone's help. These techniques could be called self-massage, or as we have called it, "Do it Yourself."

Touching yourself will bring about a feeling of intimacy and a fresh sense of your own body. With these movements you can even work on your own headache or backache. We found that many of our patients were out of touch with their own bodies, that in fact they were not even aware of certain body parts and problems in these areas. As they began to "feel" their own bodies—massaging tired feet or rubbing tired eyes—their experience was heightened by a new awareness of their sensitivities and imbalances.

Some of the techniques are easier than others, but most require little effort. As you get into these positions, simply relax and let the energy come into your hands. You will have to move or bend to reach some body parts. When there is a part that is difficult to reach, we have explained the body position required.

Heel Sit

This is one of the most powerful moves that you can do and is one of the most balancing of all techniques. It increases sexual energy, improves posture, releases tension throughout the back and neck, aids deep breathing, and stretches calf and thigh muscles. It is especially helpful for women who wear high heels and for people with general back problems.

1. Stand and spread legs about two feet apart with toes pointed at a 45-degree angle.

2. With your feet remaining flat on the floor, bend into a squatting position. *Your entire foot must remain on the floor.* If you are unable to get into a squatting position without losing your balance, either (a) lean back against a wall or (b) place a paperback book under your heels. *It is important that your weight be on your heels and not on your toes.*

3. Place elbows between your knees and clasp hands behind your head; then slowly pull your head down between your knees. You should begin to feel a tension in your upper back.

4. At the point at which the tension begins to feel uncomfortable, hold your position for about thirty seconds. Gradually increase the time until you are able to hold this position for three to five minutes.

Head Float

This technique is excellent for releasing tension in the shoulders and neck.

1. Sit in a straight-backed chair with your feet flat on the floor and your back resting against the back of the chair.

2. Imagine that you have a string attacked to the center of the top of your head with a balloon floating at the end of it. Close your eyes and visualize the balloon floating up into space, lifting your head off your neck and shoulders. If you are doing this correctly, you will actually feel your shoulders lowering and relaxing.

Scalp Tension Release

These movements help to reduce tension and headaches and also increase the health of your hair by stimulating circulation in the scalp. They also can be very helpful in revitalizing you when you are fatigued from mental effort and you still have more work to do.

1. Apply Circular Rhythmic Pressure on your scalp, using all five fingers. Do not rub

the fingers across the scalp; rather, use your fingers to move and loosen the scalp, rotating the entire hand. Rubbing the fingers is not only ineffective, but also is damaging to your hair. Also, do not work in one spot. Lift your hands and place them on different parts of the scalp. Massage the scalp for about thirty seconds.

2. Grasp a one- or two-inch thick strand of hair between your thumb and index finger, close to the scalp, and gently pull the hair. Do this for about thirty seconds. Gently tap your fingers in a "dance" all over your head for about thirty seconds.

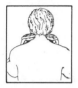

Forehead and Ear Rub

This technique, together with the eye-tension release and the nose-tension release (see below) will help to relax your facial muscles.

1. Place the palms of your hands about one-half inch apart in the center of your forehead and rub toward the center in large circular motions, applying gentle General Rhythmic Pressure. Rub six times toward the center and then six times in the opposite direction.

2. Now gently and slowly move your hands across your face toward your ears.

3. Pull the earlobes toward the shoulders. While holding this position, apply deep General Rhythmic Pressure on the lobes, using the thumb and index finger, for about one minute.

4. Now relax the lobes and, using your thumb and index finger, Muscle Knead the entire ear. The ear techniques are particularly good in helping to relax the temporal-mandibular joint, at the back of the jaw.

Eye-Tension Release

1. Using your thumb, apply firm general Rhythmic Pressure along the bone above the eye, starting at the inner corner. If you touch a particularly sensitive point, hold until the pain begins to subside.

2. Briskly rub your palms together until you begin to feel heat. With the eyes closed, place your hands over your eyes and apply gentle pressure with your palms. Hold for the count of twelve. This technique is particularly good for relaxing eye muscles and reducing eyestrain and fatigue.

Nose-Tension Release

Put thumbs into the nostrils and index fingers on the outside of the nose. Firmly pull the nose in an outward and downward direction. Do this fifteen times. This will help to open nasal passages as well as to minimize the vertical lines from the nose to the corners of the mouth.

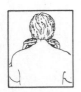

Temple-Tension Release

Place your palms above your temples, with your fingers meeting at the top of your head. Perform General Rhythmic Pressure with your palms twelve times.

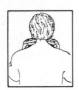

Forehead Press

1. Sit at a table or desk. Place one elbow on the table, as though you were going to arm wrestle, but with your palm facing you.

Temple-tension release: Placement of hands

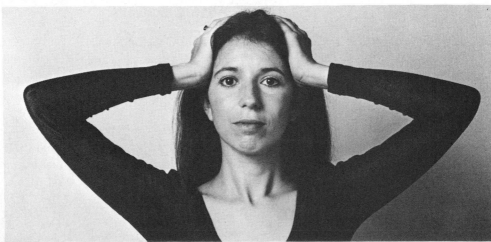

2. Lay your head in your open palm. Now apply General Rhythmic Pressure to your forehead with your palm. If you want to increase the pressure, lean your head more deeply into your hand. Do this twelve times.

Neck Squeeze

Place your hand over the back of the neck near the shoulders. Now squeeze the neck, moving from the shoulders to the point where the neck meets the head. Do this four times.

Neck squeeze: Placement of hands

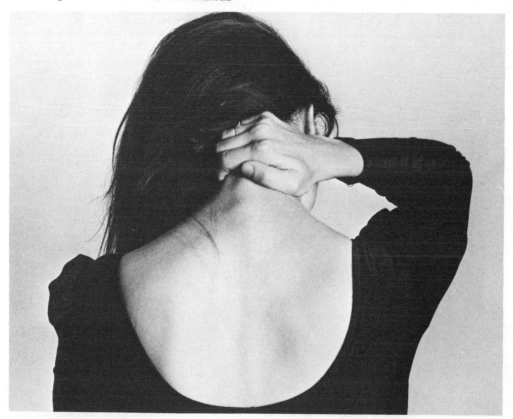

Throat Balancing

This technique relaxes throat muscles and aids in the more effective and correct use of the voice.

1. Apply very gentle General Rhythmic Pressure with your thumb and middle finger along the side of your throat. Move from the bottom of the throat to the jawbone four times.

2. Inhale and exhale deeply through mouth three times.

Shoulder-Tension Release

1. Put one hand across your chest, grasping the top of the opposite shoulder with your hand.

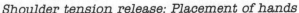

Shoulder tension release: Placement of hands

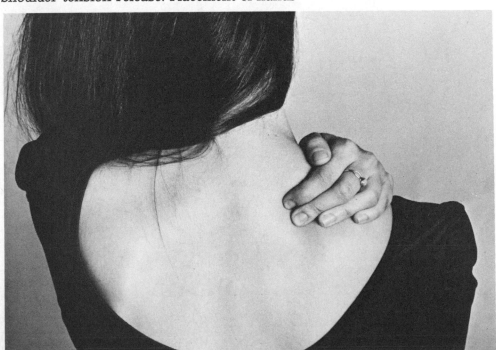

2. Perform a Muscle Squeeze on your shoulder and as far down your back as you can reach. Continue until you feel the tension leaving the area.

3. Repeat on the opposite shoulder. This will release tension in the shoulders and upper back.

4. With your arms in the same position, apply firm General Rhythmic Pressure with your middle finger from your back up to your ear.

Frontal Arm and Chest Muscle Squeeze

1. With one hand squeeze and rock the muscle to the front of your opposite armpit, holding the muscle in the web between your thumb and fingers.

2. For men only: Squeeze and rock the muscles across your chest, gripping the muscle in the palm of your hand and holding it with your thumb and fingers.

Rhythmic Pressure to Chest

Apply General Rhythmic Pressure to the chest, using all five fingers. This technique is more effective and easier when you lie flat on your back and lay your hands flat on your chest.

Arm Stretch

Extend both your arms above your head and then stretch them by "reaching for the stars." With both arms raised, stretch them one at a time, almost as though you were swimming in air. Be careful not to tense your shoulders while doing this technique. Continue for fifteen seconds.

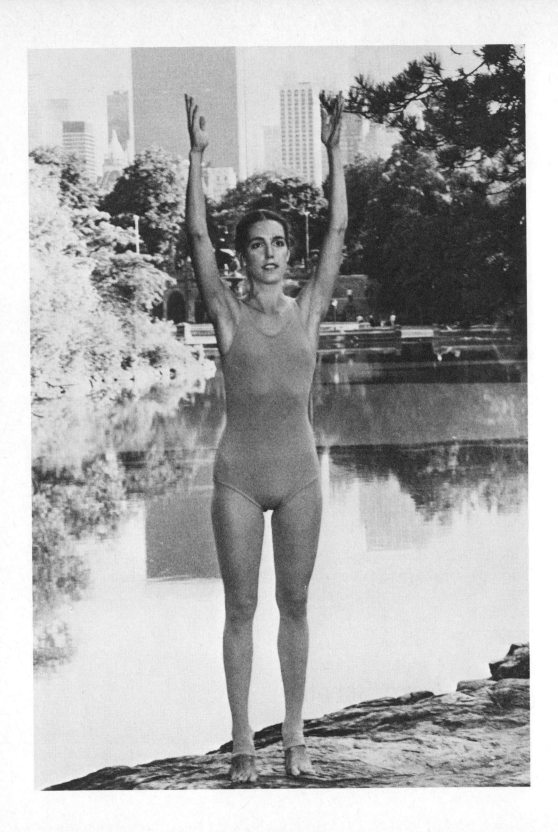

Arm Squeeze

1. Apply Muscle Squeeze to each arm, from the shoulder to the wrist.
2. Do Muscle Kneading to entire arm.
3. Repeat for the other side.

> **Caution:** *Do not apply techniques to elbows or wrists.*

Range of Motion to Elbow and Wrist

1. Support one upper arm with your other hand; extend and pull in your forearm twelve times.
2. Holding one arm just below the wrist, rotate the wrist six times clockwise and six times counterclockwise.
3. Repeat for the other side.

Leg Release

1. Sit on the floor with your legs extended in front of you. If necessary, put your back against a wall for support.
2. Perform Muscle Kneading on the top and outside of the thigh from the pelvis to the knee and to the outside of the calf from the knee to the ankle. Do it on both legs.
3. Now fold one leg across the other, resting the ankle on the knee. Do Muscle Kneading on the inside of the entire leg, from the pelvis to the ankle. Repeat for the other leg.

Abdominal Balancing

1. Lie flat on your back with your legs bent at the knees and your feet flat on the floor.

2. Gently knead the muscles around the abdomen, first clockwise and then counterclockwise.

3. Now apply General Rhythmic Pressure with your palms to the entire abdomen. These techniques will tone the entire abdominal area, vitalize the internal organs, and help eliminate constipation.

Abdominal balancing: Body position

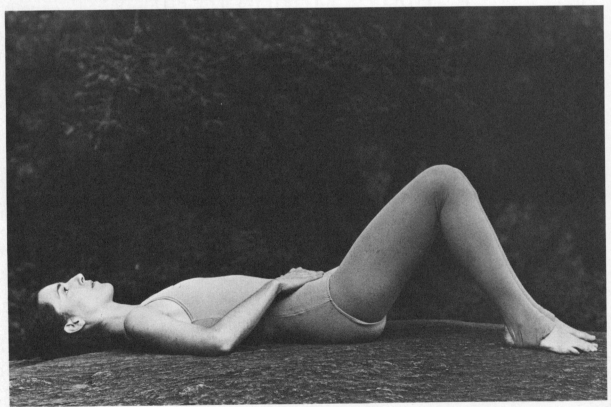

Toe Flexion

Tense all the muscles in your toes. Hold for the count of six. Release. Repeat three times.

How to flex toes

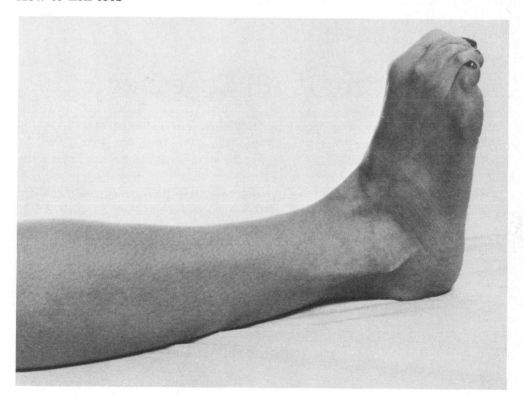

Foot Balancing

1. While sitting on the floor or on a chair, cross one ankle over the opposite knee.

2. Do a gentle Muscle Squeeze to the feet—grasp the sole of your foot in the palm of your hand and, moving from the heel to the toes, firmly squeeze the foot. Repeat for the other foot.

3. Apply General Rhythmic Pressure on feet by holding one foot in both hands with the fingers on the top of the foot and the thumbs on the sole. With the thumbs, apply firm General Rhythmic Pressure on the entire sole. Repeat for the other foot.

Putting It All Together

Now is the time again to experience your body as an entity, after having worked and concentrated on its separate parts.

1. Sit upright in a straight-backed chair, feet flat on the floor and hands resting softly on your thighs, palms down.

2. Close your eyes and relax. Make certain that your entire body, from your toes to the top of your head, is free from tension. Now visualize a lovely waterfall, a seaside, a field of daisies, a blue sky with gentle clouds—anything that you associate with peace and calm. Breathe evenly and rhythmically from your diaphragm. Rid your mind of thoughts and experience the energy flowing through your body. Stay in this quiet state until your body tells you that it's time to move.

CHAPTER 6

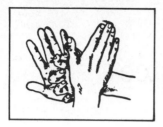

BODY PARTS THAT HURT

Do you ever wake up in the morning with every muscle in your body aching? Or you can't raise your arm? Or your lower back hurts so much, you feel as if you carried the Empire State Building around the block three times—all by yourself? Or your knees and ankles are rigid with pain? And you feel as if you were at least twenty years older than you actually are? And as you try slowly to crawl out of bed, do you wonder why this is happening to you? Why you have been so afflicted? After all, you can't remember having done anything out of the ordinary that should have put you in this miserable state.

Well, the painful truth is that you may have brought on the agony by habitually neglecting some essential rules of health care. During your lifetime you have probably developed some bad habits that are beginning to talk back to you. Aches, pains, tension, and other types of impairment usually are the body's attempt to tell you that you have been doing something wrong.

The seven basic causes of imbalances in the body are lack of exercise, poor nutrition, emotional tension, occupational stress, poor breathing patterns, incorrect posture, and injuries—all of which are discussed in other chapters in this book. This chapter will tell you how to detect specific imbalances, information on what causes them, and specific techniques for correcting them. You may perform most of these techniques on yourself. Some, however, require a partner.

The Head and Face

Signs of imbalance in the head and face:

○ Pain in any area of the head or face.
○ Problems with the temporal-mandibular joint (TMJ), which is located at the back of the jaw line, just in front of the ear. This joint moves each time the jaw opens or closes. Most people have some degree of imbalance in this area, frequently caused by emotional tension and sometimes by dental braces. Symptoms of TMJ imbalance include ringing in the ears, a painful clicking sound when chewing, headaches over the temples, difficulty opening and closing the mouth, locked jaw.
○ Squinting the eyes constantly.
○ Raising the eyebrows constantly.
○ Blinking the eyes very frequently or extremely rarely.
○ Excessive sensitivity to light or sound.
○ A tight pinched look around the mouth.
○ Grinding or clenching the teeth.
○ Biting the lips, tongue, or inside of the cheek constantly.

Causes of imbalance in the head and face:

○ Injuries to the head, neck, face, or shoulders.
○ Emotional stress and tension and negative reactions such as fear, anger, anxiety, and depression.
○ Poor circulation.
○ Air pollution, constant loud noise, excessively bright lights, cigarette smoking, and consumption of alcohol, refined sugar, pork, coffee, or chemical preservatives and food additives.
○ Occupations that require a great deal of mental activity.
○ Poor postural and other musculoskeletal imbalances.
○ Improper breathing habits and lack of exercise.

Techniques to relieve head and face imbalances:
To increase circulation and relax head muscles—

1. Headstands and shoulderstands are excellent and not as difficult as they appear (see Chapter 8). Or, use a slant board for at least five minutes twice a day. These techniques are good for the entire body and help to raise your overall energy level.

2. Lightly and rapidly tap your fingers on your forehead and top of your head as if you were dancing with your fingers or typing.

3. Apply Vital Force Contact to points along the centerline of the head from the point between the eyebrows back to the base of the skull. Hold each contact for the count of six.

4. Apply Circular Rhythmic Pressure to the neck approximately one inch below the ear. To locate the point, place a hand on each side of the head, fingers pointing toward the shoulders. Slide your hands down until the web between the thumb and index finger rests against the back of the ear. Apply light Circular Rhythmic Pressure with the index finger for about twenty seconds.

Take a one- or two-inch strand of hair between your thumb and fingers. Hold close to the scalp and pull gently. Repeat over the entire head.

These techniques not only will help to prevent or relieve headaches, but also they will help to improve your memory and increase your mental acumen and stamina.

To relieve aches in any part of the head:

1. Apply General Rhythmic Pressure on the back of the head where the neck meets the occipital bone. This must be done by a partner. (See occipital bone, page 67.) First have a partner cradle your head in the palms of his hands, with the tips of the fingers at the base of the skull. (See head cradle in Chapter 3.) Have him apply General Rhythmic Pressure on the knotty areas where the head and neck meet, using the three middle fingers on each hand. The procedure starts with simultaneously pressing the index finger on each hand. Have partner hold each finger pressure for the count of ten. Then he moves to the middle finger and finally the ring finger. Repeat the process six times. When he is finished applying General Rhythmic Pressure, he should cradle your head for about two or three minutes. This will have a very relaxing and soothing effect, which in some cases makes one feel as if the entire body is being cradled.

2. Use Range of Motion to rotate your head six times in each direction.

3. Lower your head and apply Circular Rhythmic Pressure at the back of the head around the base of the skull.

To relieve headaches in the temple area or on the sides of the head:

Apply General Rhythmic Pressure on the sides of your head immediately above the temples. First, hold your head in your hands with the base of the palms placed just above the temples and the tips of the fingers meeting on the centerline of the crown. Apply General Rhythmic Pressure with the palms; hold the pressure for the count of ten. Repeat six times. When you have finished applying General Rhythmic Pressure, continue to hold the head gently in your hands for about two or three minutes.

To relieve facial tensions and relax the temporal-mandibular joint:

1. Slowly open the jaw as wide as possible and then slowly close it. Repeat six times.

2. Slowly move jaw from side to side six times in each direction.

3. Tense all your facial muscles, puckering your lips and squinting your eyes. Hold as tightly as you can for the count of six and then release and slowly relax.

Do one of these exercises whenever you feel your facial muscles getting tense. You should do one of these exercises at least four times during the day to exercise your facial muscles and keep the TMJ relaxed.

Since TMJ problems are often caused by dental braces, we recommend that braces be used only when necessary for dental health. If you are planning to use them solely for cosmetic purposes, you should first consult with a dentist who is well trained in TMJ work, cranial manipulation, and the long-term effects of dental braces.

A special note about headaches:

Headaches can be symptomatic of a wide variety of disturbances. If they are particularly painful, persistent, or frequent, see a physician. Many headaches, however, are a result of tension, stress, or other imbalances that can be corrected with the techniques listed above and other relaxation techniques. To help prevent headaches, eat correctly (see Nutrition, Chapter 10), get plenty of fresh air and exercise, practice deep breathing, and try not to think too much or worry. When you feel a headache coming on, stop what you are doing, inhale and exhale six times slowly, drink a cup of peppermint tea, and if possible, sit or lie down in a quiet place, rest your head, close your eyes, and try to visualize a pleasant scene, such as a field of fresh flowers or a seaside.

 # The Eyes

Because they are connected to so many parts of the body, the eyes are easily affected by imbalances in other parts of the body. The eyes are particularly vulnerable to liver imbalances, which are often reflected by puffiness, darkness, and bags under the eyes. There is a theory that information about problems throughout the body can be detected through specific patterns in the iris. This practice is known as irridology. To protect the health of your eyes, make certain that you have sufficient intake of vitamin A and get plenty of fresh air, since the eyes need a large oxygen intake in order to function properly. Your eyes are very delicate, and any persistent problem should be checked by a qualified health-care professional.

To strengthen muscles in the eyes and relieve eyestrain:

1. Place your open hands on a table, palms up. Close your eyes and rest your eyes on your palms, with the center of your palms placing a light pressure on your eyes. Hold for a count of thirty.

2. Close your eyes tight and tense the muscles. Now stretch your arms over your head, pushing as high as you can, and make tight fists. Hold for a count of ten. Now slowly relax your eyes and lower your arms.

3. Perform Range of Motion: Without moving your head, look as far to the left as you can. Return to center. Then look as far as you can to the right. Return to center. Now look down to the tip of your nose, return to center, and look up as high as you can. You may want to use your fingers as a guide, holding your arms at shoulder height, with a finger pointed to the left and right, and then above and slightly to the front of your head when looking up. Hold each eye position for a count of ten.

The Sinuses

To relieve sinus pain and congestion:

1. Perform a continuous Muscle Squeeze on the tips of the fingers and toes, which are reflex points for the sinuses. Squeeze each for about thirty seconds.

2. Apply General Rhythmic Pressure to the corner of each nostril.

3. Decrease intake of mucus-producing foods such as cheese, milk, and all junk foods. Get plenty of fresh air and exercise. Use a room humidifier to keep the air moist.

The Teeth

To relieve toothache pain:

1. Gently apply General Rhythmic Pressure to the entire jaw. Hold each pressure point for about fifteen seconds.

2. Apply Vital Force Contact to the points on either side of the ear. (See Vital Force Contact Points Chart, Chapter 3.) These techniques will help provide temporary relief until you can see a dentist.

The Neck and Throat

Signs of imbalance in the neck and throat:

○ Limited range of motion in the neck.
○ Exaggerated tilt of the neck to one side (torticollis).
○ Inability to touch chest with chin.
○ Bulging veins in the neck.
○ Tension headaches.
○ Grinding the teeth (bruxism).
○ Imbalances in the shoulders.
○ Difficulty in breathing.
○ Chronic sore throat.
○ High-pitched voice, inability to project the voice, chronic hoarseness.
○ Chronic coughing or tics in the throat.

What your voice says about you:

Your voice reflects your emotional state because your emotional state affects your sound-producing organs. The voice is a delicate yet powerful instrument that is used continually by most people. It can go from a whisper to a roar. The way you use it—the tone, pitch, timbre, expression, loudness or softness—determines to a very large extent the impact you have on others, especially in that very important first encounter. People tend to read your personality and character from your voice and to react accordingly. A well-pitched and modulated voice connotes control, self-assurance, and authority to the listener.

When you habitually hold back strong feelings and thoughts out of excessive defer-ence, fear, or anxiety, the larynx and throat muscles become tight and constricted. It is not unusual, for example, to hear someone say that the words he wanted to express got "stuck" in his throat. This is often more literal than we think and can result in a chronic mild soreness or what seems like a tic in the throat. On the other hand, people who talk excessively, speaking before they think, are likely to stretch and strain the voice and develop a chronic hoarseness. Professionals who use their voice as their primary tool, such as lawyers, singers, teachers, and television or radio announcers, are prime candi-dates for imbalances in the throat area, especially when they have never learned how to project their voices properly.

Causes of imbalance in the neck and throat:

○ Chronic tension in neck due to emotional factors.
○ Chronic tension in throat and neck muscles caused by poor speaking or vocal habits.
○ Inhibitions in saying what you think and feel.
○ Smoking.
○ Eating mucus-producing foods that coat and block the throat, limiting vocal range and endurance. Different foods produce mucus in different people, but more often than not dairy products, wheat, and meat are the biggest culprits.
○ Shock to the neck such as whiplash and other injuries.
○ Occupations that require the neck to be held in one position for extended periods of time, such as dentistry, modeling, typing, writing.
○ Poor posture.
○ Carrying a heavy bag or pocketbook on one shoulder constantly.
○ General tension in upper back.
○ Overweight.
○ Poorly fitted or high-heeled shoes.
○ Congenital contraction in neck or upper back muscles.
○ Incorrect sleeping habits such as sleeping on your stomach, sleeping with arms or hands under your neck or head, sleeping on a mattress that is too soft.

Techniques for relieving neck and throat imbalances:

To relax throat and neck muscles and release blockages:

1. Apply gentle Vital Force Contact on the back of the neck and gently over the throat.

2. Use Range of Motion to rotate head and neck six times clockwise and six times counterclockwise.

3. The Yoga lion brings results both in toning and relaxing muscles and clearing the throat. Open your mouth as wide as possible, tense all your facial muscles, and stick your tongue out as far as possible. Hold for the count of six.

4. Hum the sound *ōoooommmmmm*. Project the sound deep into your throat. Then make the sound *ēeeeeeăaaaaa* deep in your throat. Repeat the sequence three times. In both cases you should feel the vibrations deep in your throat. This helps to renew and strengthen the voice and throat.

5. Use a warm-water compress on your throat to relax tight muscles (see page 110, "Throat Balancing").

To reduce pain, inflammation, and congestion from a sore throat and increase circulation to the area:

1. Apply penetrating oils, such as Olbas, Tiger Balm, or peppermint, which are

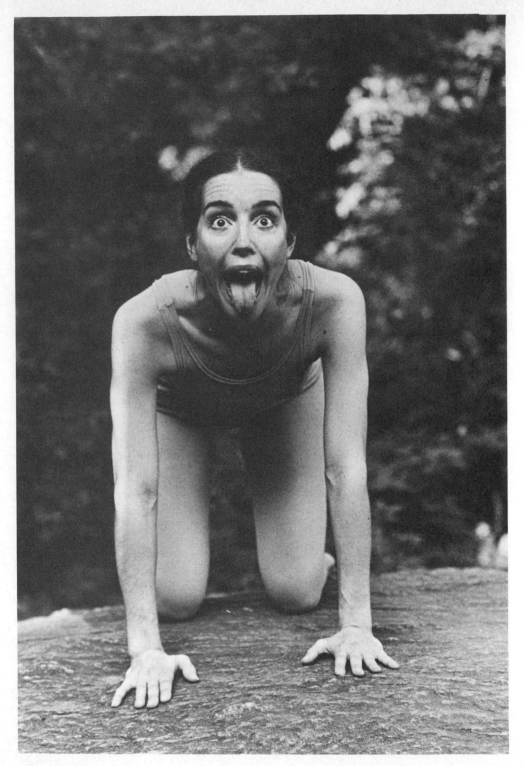

Yoga Lion

available in health-food stores. First apply oil to a moist, lukewarm cloth. Wrap the cloth around the throat as you would a compress. Leave it on overnight.

> **Caution:** *Do not apply over open sores, abrasions, or cuts. This can be very painful and irritating.*

2. Gargle with a warm salt-water solution: 1 teaspoon of salt to 6 ounces of water.
3. To help prevent throat problems, use a mixture of honey, warm water, and lemon before and after using your voice for an extended period. Also, be certain to protect your throat with a scarf or collar during winter months.

> **Caution:** *If a sore throat persists, obtain professional medical advice. Sore throats can be connected with and lead to serious complications.*

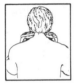

The Shoulders

Signs of imbalance in the shoulders:

- Chest pushed forward.
- Rounded shoulders.
- One shoulder higher than the other.
- One shoulder shorter than the other.
- Imbalance in the hip joint.

Causes of imbalance in the shoulders:

- Poor posture.
- Occupations that require the shoulders to be held in one position for extended periods of time (e.g., typing, modeling, certain types of assembly-line work).
- Prolonged tension in the upper back, often related to emotional stress or high pressure work. Chronic doubt and confusion are indicated by tension in the shoulders, often shown by hunched, raised shoulders.
- Worktables and desks that are too high. This will cause you to raise

your shoulders, bringing tightness and pain. To determine proper table height, bend your elbows when you are in a sitting position. The table should be even with your elbows.

○ Carrying a heavy bag on one shoulder. This is especially common among dancers and women.

○ Poor breathing habits. Shoulder tension will be released more easily as you learn to breathe from your diaphragm.

○ Overweight.

○ Accidents that cause a violent contraction of shoulder muscles.

○ Shock to the neck, such as whiplash or other injuries.

Techniques for relieving shoulder imbalances:

To release deep-rooted emotional inhibitions reflected in the shoulders and upper back and assist breathing and digestion:

Use Circular Rhythmic Pressure around the inside border of the shoulder blades.

To relax the muscles and prepare them for further bodywork:

1. Apply a penetrating oil (Olsa, Tiger Balm, peppermint) directly on the shoulder area and massage gently into skin. Place a moist, warm compress on the area for about twenty minutes; do not make it too hot.

2. Have Muscle Rock performed on shoulders and upper back while you are lying on your stomach.

To improve circulation, stretch and tonify the muscles near the shoulders:

1. Use Muscle Kneading on shoulders.

To strengthen the flow of energy and relieve muscle tension:

1. Apply Circular or General Rhythmic Pressure to the shoulders.

2. Apply Law of Similars Contacts on the buttocks and shoulder blades.

Use massage techniques for the shoulders, given in Chapter 4, "Doing a Full Massage Session," page 97.

(See Shoulder-Tension Release, page 110.)

 # The Arms and Hands

Signs of imbalance in the arms and hands:

○ One shoulder higher than the other.

○ Chest pushed forward.

○ Rounded shoulders.

○ Constant knuckle cracking.
○ Constant finger twitching.
○ Cold hands and/or arms.
○ Abnormally sweaty hands.
○ Constant folding of arms across the chest.
○ Inability to make grasping motions with fingers.
○ Pain in the hand when trying to grip something.
○ Swollen fingers.

Causes of imbalance in the arms and hands:

○ Trauma, such as surgery, or a blow to the arm or hands, or falling on outstretched hands. This can cause a fracture or dislocation of the wrist or elbow (one of the most common injuries among rollerskaters or ice skaters).
○ Improper gripping of a tennis racket or a tool. This can irritate the bursas (closed, fluid-filled sacs usually found between tendons and bones in areas subject to friction such as shoulders and elbows).
○ Excessive strain on the wrist joint. This is commonly experienced by weight lifters who attempt to do certain curls improperly.
○ Hyperextension of the elbow. This is common in weight lifters and gymnasts.
○ Rheumatoid arthritis can result in severe limitation of elbow motion.
○ Osteoarthritis may limit the range of motion and cause stiffness and inflammation in muscles and joints.
○ Professions that require precision work with the hands (e.g., sewing, fine jewelry work, electronics, typing).
○ Arthritic conditions.

People who have problems in their ankles tend to have problems in their wrists; problems in knees are usually reflected in elbows; and problems in toes are often reflected in fingers. (See "Law of Similars," page 64.)

Techniques for relieving arm and hand imbalances:

To increase circulation, to bring nutrients to the hands, to remove cellular waste from the hands, and to increase the flow of energy, alternate hot and cold hand soaks. Prepare two pans of water, approximately three quarts each, one hot and one cold. The hot water should be approximately 106 degrees, the cold approximately 40 degrees. Place hands first in the hot water for about two minutes. Then place them in the cold water for about fifteen seconds. Repeat process three times. Always begin with hot water and finish with cold.

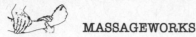

> *Caution:* Do not use hot water when there is inflammation.

To correct general imbalances and increase movement in the wrist, hands, and fingers, use firm General Rhythmic Pressure and Muscle Kneading on the muscles of the lower arm.

To correct general imbalances in the wrist after surgery, use Muscle Kneading not only on the wrist, but on the entire arm.

> *Caution:* Check first with surgeon.

To correct general imbalances in the arm and hands use Muscle Kneading on the neck on the same side where the problem is felt in the arms and hands.

To reduce muscle aches and cramps in the hands use Muscle Kneading on the forearm, palm of hand, and each finger.

To correct tennis elbow requires developing strength, flexibility, and endurance in your forearms and shoulders as well as your elbow.

1. Apply an ice pack to the elbow, ten minutes on and five minutes off.

2. Use Range of Motion to gently rotate your wrist twelve times clockwise and twelve times counterclockwise. Two other Range of Motion exercises are helpful: Place your wrist on a table about two inches in from the edge, palm facing down. Now raise your hand up and down, using the greatest range of motion. A similar Range of Motion exercise is to place your wrist on the table, palm up, and repeat the up-and-down movement. Do each exercise three times a day, performing twenty-five lifts each time. These Range of Motion exercises will help correct the elbow problem by developing the supporting muscles in the forearm.

3. Apply General Rhythmic Pressure to the area around the elbow for about three minutes several times a day.

To relieve arthritic conditions:

1. Use Range of Motion on finger joints, wrists, and elbows.

2. Apply General Rhythmic Pressure to the area around the problem joints.

The Chest

Signs of imbalance in the chest:

○ Upper back pain.
○ Respiratory problems, especially asthma, bronchitis, emphysema.
○ Shallow breathing from the chest rather than the diaphragm or lower abdomen.
○ Chest pains.
○ Heart palpitations.
○ Lumps in the breast.
○ Protruding chest.
○ Obvious imbalance in rib structure, with one side protruding more than the other.
○ Mucus buildup.

Causes of imbalance in the chest:

○ Improper breathing.
○ Smoking.
○ Air pollution.
○ Poor athletic training and techniques. (Runners often have hyperexpanded lungs that may enlarge and cause problems in the chest area.)
○ Holding the hips in one position while twisting the upper torso in the opposite direction. (This is known as rib strain and is found particularly among dancers, wrestlers, and gymnasts.)

Techniques for relieving chest imbalances:

To improve breathing, practice the correct breathing techniques given in Chapter 8, page 163.

To relax the upper back muscles use the techniques for upper and middle back given in Chapter 4, page 81.

To balance the rib cage use General Rhythmic Pressure between ribs. Move from the breastbone toward the sides. Work firmly but not too deeply.

To relax muscles in chest area and improve respiration (especially beneficial for people with asthma and other respiratory problems):

1. Use firm General Rhythmic Pressure on a line one inch below the collarbone, directly above the nipple.

2. Perform Muscle Rock on entire chest area.

3. Do deep-breathing exercises, get plenty of fresh air, sleep on your back instead of your stomach, and use a room humidifier to reduce buildup of mucus in the chest.

The Back

Signs of imbalance in the back:

- Neck tilted to one side.
- Hunched shoulders.
- Pain in back.
- Pain in chest.
- Pain in abdomen.
- Curved spine.
- Tight hamstrings or leg muscles.
- Walking on the outer or inner edge of the foot.

Causes of imbalance in the back:

- Worktables and desks that are too high. This will cause you to raise your shoulders, bringing tightness and pain. To determine proper table height, bend your elbows when you are in a sitting position. The table should be even with your elbows.
- Disk problems. If pain in the lower back has existed for some time, is fairly constant, and is very sharp, it may be the result of a rupture or disintegration of the disk.

> *Caution:* *If this is the case, it definitely should not be self-treated. See a skilled orthopedist, chiropractor, or osteopath with experience working on disk problems.*

- Poor athletic or dance training.
- Poor posture, especially when lifting heavy objects.
- Working in a sitting position for extended periods. This can tighten hamstrings and calf muscles and cause severe chronic backache.
- Malfunction or infection of any internal organs such as the kidney, liver, or pancreas.
- Infections in the spinal structure, especially in the disk spaces.
- Fractures or dislocations, especially to the vertebrae.

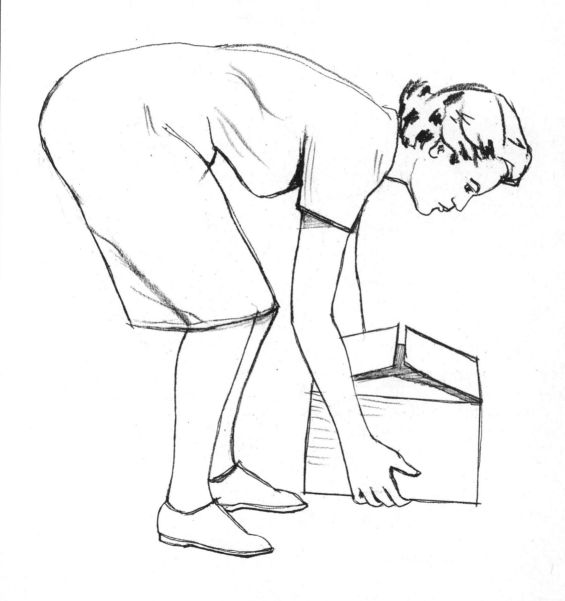

Lifting incorrectly

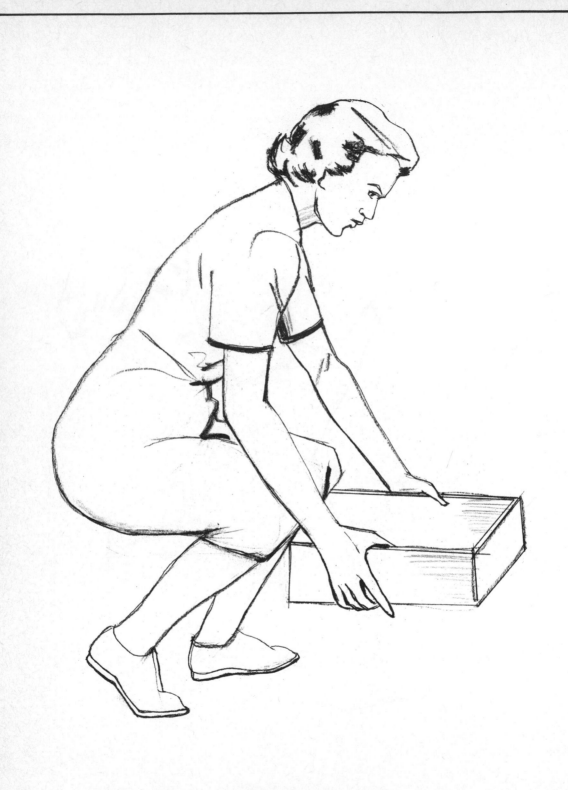

Lifting correctly

○ Bone diseases, including osteoporosis (often caused by the use of
corticosteroid drugs used to treat arthritis) and osteomalacia (softening
of the bones caused by vitamin D deficiency in an adult).
○ Imbalances in other body parts and organs, especially the abdomen,
uterus, ovaries, fallopian tubes, and prostate gland.
○ Wearing high heels.
○ Abnormal curvature of the spine (kyphosis, lordosis, scoliosis).

Techniques for relieving back imbalances:
1. Strengthen abdominal muscles by doing diaphragmatic breathing exercises. (See
"Breathing," page 216.)
2. Strengthen gluteal muscles (buttocks) to reduce stress on the back.

Leg extension to strengthen back

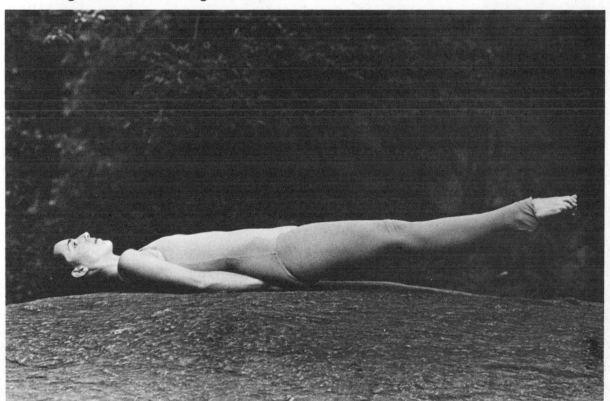

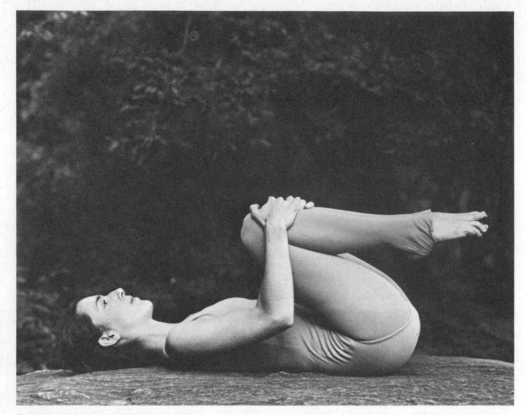

Leg hug to strengthen back

3. Strengthen lower back with the following three exercises:

Lie flat on your back with your legs extended straight in front of you. Slowly bend your knees and pull them toward your chest. Now clasp your hands on your knees and rock slowly backward and forward, hugging your knees as closely to your chest as you can. If in any position you feel tension in the part of your back where you are having difficulty, hold that position for a minute and take a deep breath and then exhale slowly while visualizing a soothing feeling penetrating the area of discomfort.

The Yoga cobra position is helpful. Lie flat on your stomach with your palms and elbows on the floor in front of you. Inhale deeply and lift your upper torso from the floor with your arms while moving your head back. As you slowly exhale, return slowly to the original position. Repeat six times.

134

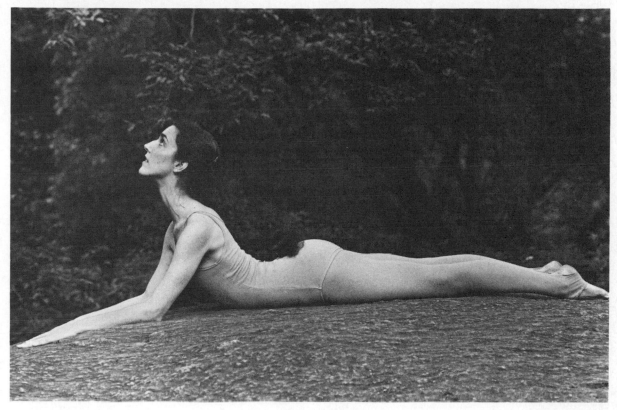

Yoga Cobra

Sit on the floor with your legs straight in front of you and your back straight. Raise your arms to shoulder height and slowly reach for your toes with your fingers. Hold for the count of three and then straighten. Repeat six times.

4. Strengthen upper and middle back with the following exercises:

To strengthen the trapezius muscle, which raises and lowers the shoulder and pulls the head backward, place your right hand *over* your right shoulder and across your back and your left hand *under* your left shoulder. Now try to "hold hands." Hold for the count of twelve. The first time you try this you may only be able to touch the tips of your index fingers. Eventually you should be able to clasp one hand in the other.

Use Range of Motion for your shoulders. Stretch your arms out at the sides at shoulder height. Make small circles and gradually increase their size. Do six clockwise

135

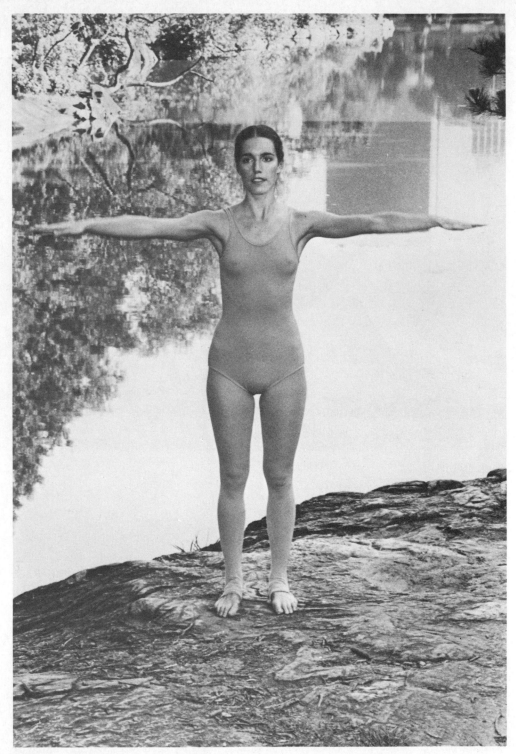

Range of Motion for shoulders

and six counterclockwise. *Or:* Lift your right shoulder toward your head and rotate it six times clockwise and six times counterclockwise. Now repeat with the left shoulder.

Use Range of Motion for your neck and thoracic vertebrae. While lying flat on your back turn your head as far as it will go to the right. Repeat three times. Now do the same thing to the left.

5. Relieve lower back pain using Range of Motion, rotating the entire leg from the hip. Do this while standing and supporting yourself against a table or the back of a chair.

6. Relieve upper back pain using Range of Motion with the head and neck, shoulders and arms.

7. Relieve upper- or lower-back pain by alternating ice massage with firm Circular Rhythmic Pressure. Place one or two ice cubes in a thick terry-cloth towel or wool flannel cloth or an ice bag and place directly on skin for fifteen to thirty seconds. Then apply Circular Rhythmic Pressure on the area.

Caution: Do not use ice over the kidneys or do bodywork too deeply in this area.

A special note on back problems

To prevent back problems, be careful how you reach and bend to pick up heavy objects, and watch your posture when you are sitting to make certain that your back and spine are well supported. Always try to be aware of your posture, whether you are sitting or standing.

Avoid excessive bed rest. This will cause atrophy of the muscles in the lower back and abdomen and also lead to osteoporosis and further muscle spasms.

Use alternating hot and cold showers daily, with a strong spray on areas of tension and pain.

Use cool to lukewarm packs, Epsom salt, or compresses on the area of discomfort.

Occasionally the imbalance in the back may be so great that a back brace or orthopedic corset may be required to give adequate support to the lower thoracic and lumbar spine as well as to the abdominal muscles. This should be determined by a health professional trained in making such evaluations.

The Abdomen

Signs of imbalance in the abdomen:

○ Poor muscle tone in abdomen, lower back, and leg muscles.
○ Uneven distribution of body weight when standing (greater weight on one leg or hip).
○ Pelvis extended forward.
○ Tight buttocks.
○ Constipation.
○ Lower-back pain.
○ Extremely tight front and back thigh muscles.
○ Digestive problems.
○ Flatulence and stomach cramps.
○ Menstrual cramps.

Causes of imbalance in the abdomen:

○ Poor posture.
○ Congenital weakness.
○ Lack of exercise.
○ Tight clothes, such as girdles, tight belts, and tight jeans, tend to restrict the motion of the abdominal muscles as well as the muscles of the lower back. In addition, they affect breathing by restricting the proper action of the diaphragm.
○ Diseases of the abdomen, such as stomach cancer, ulcers, internal-organ (e.g., kidney, liver) malfunctions, hemorrhoids.
○ Gas trapped in abdomen and rib cage.
○ Imbalances in the digestive system.
○ Incorrect use of back muscles, such as picking up heavy objects incorrectly.
○ Pregnancy.
○ Repressed emotions such as anger, fear, and jealousy.

Techniques for relieving abdominal imbalances:
1. Release blockages by applying light General Rhythmic Pressure on the points two

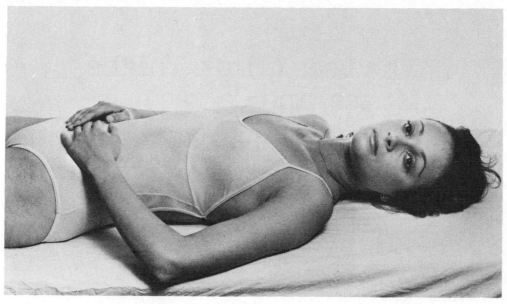

Applying General Rhythmic Pressure for abdominal imbalances

inches on either side of the navel. Follow with medium Circular Rhythmic Pressure on the lower back, directly behind the navel.

2. Tone intestinal muscles and help eliminate waste by applying circular Rhythmic Pressure to the entire abdomen in a clockwise direction, using heel of the hand rather than the thumb. *Caution: If there is suspected pregnancy, acute pain, or any organ malfunction, do not use this technique or any other form of deep pressure.*

3. Increase bowel regularity by increasing fiber content and decreasing refined foods in your diet. Also, apply gentle Vital Force Contact one inch below the navel. Apply pressure three times for fifteen seconds each time.

4. Release and soothe repressed emotions by doing relaxation and deep breathing exercises.

5. Relieve gas pains and menstrual cramps by performing Muscle Rock on the abdomen.

6. Strengthen abdominal muscles by doing the Yoga cobra (see page 134) and situps. Lie on your back with your knees bent and your feet flat on the floor. With your hands locked at the base of your head, lift your trunk until the elbows touch your knees. Hold for the count of six. Slowly lower your back to the floor, one vertebra at a time. Repeat six times.

The Legs (Hips, Thighs, Knees, and Calves)

Signs of imbalance in the legs:

O Pain in lower back.
O Pelvic area protrudes forward.
O Tightness in front or back of thighs.
O Very bulky, muscular thighs.
O Locked knee joint.
O Difficulty bending knee.
O Pain in knee. If pain is on the outside of the knee, the primary imbalance is on the inside of the thigh and shin. If the pain is on the back of the knee, the primary imbalance is probably in the calf muscles and the hamstring.

Caution: Pain under the knee cap or a knee that is unable to bend or straighten completely may be an indication of torn cartilage and may require professional attention.

O Walking with a limp when there is no medical reason.
O Difficulty kneeling or sitting "Japanese style," with legs folded under the body.
O Chronic pain in calf or thigh muscles.
O Inability to stand for long periods of time.
O Stiffness in hip joints, particularly after sitting for a period of time.
O Knock knees or bow legs.

Causes of imbalance in legs:

O Congenital structural defects such as knock knees, pigeon toes, or bowed legs.

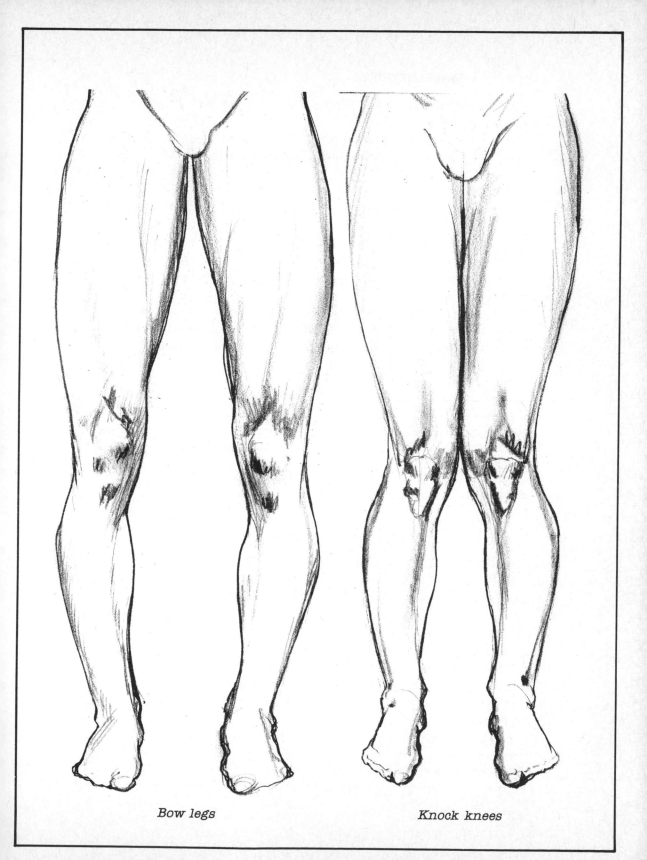

Bow legs   *Knock knees*

o Structural imbalances such as calcium deposits, bone spurs, or excess fluid in the joints.
o One leg that is shorter than the other.
o Injuries to the ankle, the most common being a sprain.
o Overweight.
o Pregnancy.
o Constant kneeling and bruising over a long period of time may irritate the bursas under the knee. This is commonly called "housewife's knee" and can be prevented by wearing knee pads.
o Injuries to the knee. Of particular concern are meniscus injuries, which involve injury to the crescent-shaped cartilage in the knee joint. Because this type of injury is most commonly found among football players, it is often called "football knee." It can result from a blow to the outside of the knee or a forced sideways bending of the knee joint (which the knee is not designed for) caused by stepping in a hole or any motion that turns the ankle.

> *Caution: This injury requires professional attention, however, our bodywork for knee imbalances is often helpful.*

o Shin splints. These can result from either the tearing of a membrane between the two shin bones or the tearing of a muscle in the shins.
o Arthritic conditions.

Techniques for relieving leg imbalances:

1. Prevent shin splints by applying deep Circular and General Rhythmic Pressure on the shins between the two lower leg bones. Then use Range of Motion on ankle, moving the foot up and down thirty-six times. Correct shin splints by sitting with the leg elevated as much as possible, applying Circular Rhythmic Pressure on shin, rubbing an ice bag up and down shins, five minutes on and five minutes off, for thirty minutes.

2. Relieve congested muscles, relax tight muscles, and increase circulation for the entire leg by applying deep General Rhythmic Pressure using the palm of the hand down the entire leg, working on the front, back and side of the thigh and the back and side of the calf.

> *Caution: Do not press on knee and do not press on shinbone.*

Follow with Muscle Kneading on the entire leg, working on the front, back, and side of the thigh and the back and side of the calf.

> **Caution:** *Do not work on knee or on shinbone.*

3. Strengthen the energy flow in the lower leg by applying Law of Similars, making contact with the hip and shoulder and the knee and elbow (on the same side of the body).

4. Strengthen the energy flow in the thigh, by using the Muscle Rock. Place one hand on the sensitive point about one-half to one inch on the inside of the pelvic bone. With the other hand, grasp the thigh firmly, without squeezing too hard, and begin to rock thigh muscles from side to side while pressing firmly but not too deeply on pelvic point.

5. After an injury, use the following methods to strengthen the knee:

Muscle Rock to the thigh

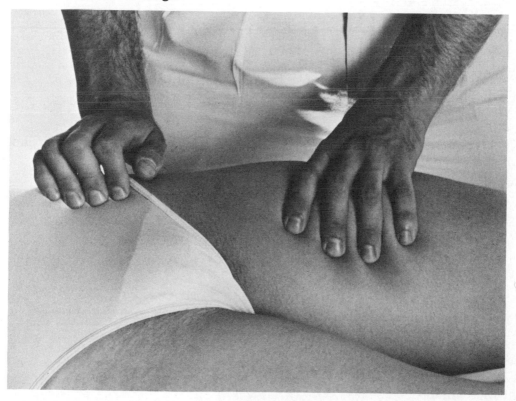

For the first twenty-four hours, use an elastic brace on the knee whenever leg is in use. However, try to stay off the leg as much as possible.

For most minor injuries to the knee, apply cold water or ice packs for twenty-four hours, stay off the leg, and elevate the knee. When using ice or cold water packs, apply for twenty minutes and then remove for fifteen. After ice packs have been used for twenty-four hours, apply warm castor-oil packs. (See Chapter 9.) (Some people have reported positive results from DMSO, a waste product of the wood pulp industry. There have been claims of therapeutic benefit from its use, particularly in cases where surgery seemed to be the only course of action.)

Flex, or contract, the thigh muscle against the hand. This strengthens the quadriceps muscles, which stabilize the knees.

Use Arnica lotion, available in health-food stores, in a manner similar to penetrating oils (see page 123).

Many knee injuries incurred today are the result of poor running and jogging habits, the worst of which is wearing poorly designed and poorly fitted shoes. To prevent knee injuries, if you run or jog, even occasionally, you should invest in a good pair of runner's shoes.

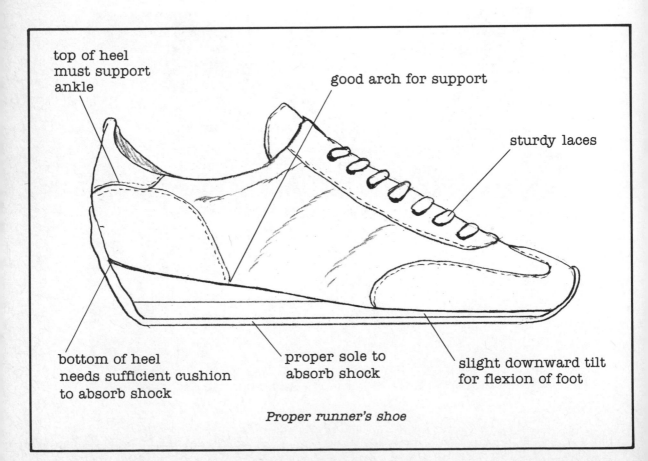

Proper runner's shoe

> **_Caution_** _for runners with knee problems: Do not exert any pressure on the knee or do exercises that cause you to bend your leg._

6. Strengthen the calf muscles and the Achilles tendon:

Perform Range of Motion with your foot. This is most effective if done while lying on your back. Lift the foot five to ten inches off the floor and rotate it six times clockwise and six times counterclockwise.

Stand approximately three feet from a wall, facing it, and rest your hands on the wall. Make certain that your body is on an angle. Now slowly raise your heels until you are standing on your toes. Hold this position for a count of twenty and then slowly lower your heels to the ground. Repeat three times.

Do the Muscle Rock, followed by Circular Rhythmic Pressure, on your calf.

The Ankles and Feet

Signs of imbalance in the ankles and feet:

○ Hammertoe, a condition in which the first bone of the toe points upward while the second and third bones point downward.
○ Toe joints that are constantly flexed, usually due to tension and contracted hamstrings.
○ Flat feet (fallen arches). People with this imbalance usually wear out the inner edges of the soles of their shoes.
○ High instep (high arch).
○ Extreme sensitivity to touch. This may be experienced as ticklishness, pain, or a general dislike of having the feet touched.
○ Feet turned extremely in or out, "pigeon toed" or "slew-footed." (Slew footedness, excessive turnout of the foot and ankle, and the resultant tension in the foot, ankle, and knee is commonly experienced by ballet dancers who have been improperly trained.)
○ Hip and splint problems.

Causes of imbalance in the ankles and feet:

○ Pointed or poorly fitted shoes. These place the foot in a bind similar to that of a splint, which causes the ligaments to shorten, the joint capsules to contract, adhesions to form where they should not be, and an increasingly rigid longitudinal arch that can affect the structural balance of the entire body. More often than not, misshaped toes are due to poor shoe choice over the years.

○ A rotated pelvis may result in fallen arches.

○ Tightness of inner-thigh and lower-back muscles may result in fallen arches, although in many cases, fallen arches are congenital.

○ High insteps. This places the body's center of gravity in the wrong place, and can cause extensive postural problems.

○ Compression of the nerve against the thighbone, crossing the legs, and wearing high heels can contribute to a condition known as "dropped foot." This is an abnormal extension, or movement of the top of the foot away from the shinbone. When a person is wearing high heels, the foot is in a state of abnormal extension (or plantar flexion).

○ Poor posture when walking.

○ Standing on your feet for extended periods of time.

Techniques for relieving ankle and foot imbalances:

Treatment of the feet has four primary goals—to improve circulation around the feet, to stabilize the position of the feet in relation to the legs so that the body is correctly balanced, to create a full range of motion for all joints of the foot, and to strengthen the supporting muscles in the foot. To achieve these four basic goals, the following techniques are recommended:

1. Range of Motion on feet. Rotate each foot twelve times clockwise and counterclockwise.

2. Range of Motion on toes. Grasp the tip of each toe and rotate clockwise three times and counterclockwise three times.

3. Flex the foot three times upward (toward shinbone) and three times downward (away from shinbone).

4. Law of Similars Contact on ankles and wrists; toes and fingers.

5. Twice a day, elevate the feet for five to ten minutes.

6. Tap the bottom of the feet with fingertips in a very rapid motion. This has a tonifying effect. (See chart on foot reflexology, page 23.)

7. Use gentle General Rhythmic Pressure along the outsides of the feet.

8. Muscle Squeeze the calf and the feet.

9. Soak ankles and feet in warm water with Epsom salts or sea salt.

To help correct a sprained ankle, after first aid has been applied:

1. Immediately after the sprain, apply an ice bag or a cold-water compress. Apply for 15 minutes every hour. Continue for twenty-four hours.

2. After twenty four hours, begin to do Range of Motion exercises. Use only up-and-

down movements in the beginning. While standing on one foot, lift your sprained ankle from the floor about twelve inches and then slowly point your toe down and then up. Proceed through this movement six times. Repeat several times a day. After this, you can begin to do circular Range of Motion.

3. Whenever possible, elevate the foot. This will revitalize the area.

4. Twenty-four hours after the sprain, soak your foot in a solution of Epsom salts.

5. When the pain and swelling begin to subside, apply circular Rhythmic Pressure to the entire area around the ankle.

6. After two or three days, while standing, lift the right heel slowly and shift the weight to the left foot. Then slowly lift your right heel and shift your weight to the right foot while lowering it to the floor. Keep your toes on the floor at all times. Repeat six times for each foot.

Tension, Hypertension, Impotence

In addition to relieving the musculoskeletal imbalances that we have discussed, our techniques have proved to be beneficial in other common types of imbalances, three of which are tension, hypertension (high blood pressure) and impotence.

Tension

Signs of tension:

- Furrowed eyebrows and/or lines on forehead.
- Headache.
- Insomnia.
- Grinding of teeth (bruxism).
- Squinting eyes.
- Backaches.
- Tight shoulders.

Causes of tension:

○ Stressful occupation. Tension at the work place can accumulate and lead to physical illness.

○ Poor sleeping habits. The cause can be improper mattress, too many pillows, street noises, ingestion of a heavy meal or snacks at bedtime, and not enough fresh air. Lack of certain vitamins, especially B6, may prevent the achievement of certain brain rhythms so that the deep sleep period is not entered.

○ Nutritional deficiencies. Diet deficient in essential vitamins and minerals.

○ Poor posture. Incorrect body alignment places undue stress on all parts of the body.

○ No outlet for emotional expression. All work and no play does more than make Jack or Jane dull.

○ Lack of exercise. Physical exercise—whether it is jogging around the park or in place in your apartment—is the best way to relieve tension. Exercise is a necessary part of the daily "rat race," and even at your place of work, an exercise break can be better for increasing your efficiency level than a coffee break.

Techniques to Relieve Tension:

1. Apply General Rhythmic Pressure to the back of the head using the flat area of the thumbs. Begin at the back of the head where it joins the neck (occiput area). Lightly press this area all the way across from left to right, then from right to left. Apply pressure to the entire surface at least three times before moving to the next area.

2. Next knead the ears. Place the ear lobe between the thumb and the index finger and with a rubbing motion, softly squeeze. Repeat several times on each ear.

3. Muscle Rock the stomach. The receiver should lie flat on his back. Place one hand on the lower abdomen and the other hand directly on the stomach. Rock the stomach with a gentle back and forth motion.

4. Apply Rhythmic Pressure to the feet (see page 94).

5. Muscle Rock the back (see page 82).

6. Finish with a visualization, used as a progressive relaxation exercise. Ask the receiver to lie flat on his back. He should slowly close his eyes, take a slow, deep breath, inhale, hold it, and release. Repeat this three times.

Next ask him to visualize a soft blue sky with white fluffy clouds gently passing over head. He must let his entire body go limp. Tell him, "Take the tension first from your feet by contracting the muscles. Now totally release and relax." Repeat this process, this time asking him to tense the front and back leg muscles. Repeat this three times, tensing then releasing.

Ask him to shrug his shoulders, make a fist, and then release and relax. Finally tense the face, pucker the lips, tightly close the eyes, and then release. Relax and release. Now tell him to take another deep breath and exhale, allowing his total body to relax.

Hypertension

Hypertension is often related to emotional stress, poor nutritional habits, or lack of exercise. Specific factors related to hypertension include overeating, too much refined sugar, too much salt in the diet, excessive smoking, excessive alcohol consumption, poor emotional disposition, and kidney dysfunction. In addition to watching your diet and getting plenty of exercise, various relaxation techniques can be of benefit in controlling hypertension. We suggest a gentle Muscle Rock on the stomach area to strengthen the kidneys, daily relaxation and visualization exercises, and a weekly full body massage to help soothe and relax the nervous system and revitalize the vital organs.

Impotence

Most men experience impotence at some time in their lives. It can result from emotional or physical problems or a combination of both. Research indicates that in fifty percent of the cases impotence is caused by psychological factors. Many cases with a physical basis are related to the use of medication, including those that are often prescribed for hypertension. If the impotence is prolonged, see a qualified urologist, since there are many new methods for treating both psychological and physical impotence. If the problem is psychological, and even in some cases where there is a physical basis, it is important to learn to relax and rid the body of negative emotions such as fear, worry, hate, and jealousy. Also recommended are techniques that help to energize and revitalize the system, such as headstands, shoulder stands, or the use of a slant board for at least five minutes a day. General imbalances in sexual energy, such as premature ejaculation, loss of erection, frigidity, and diminished sexual drive, may be corrected by the use of herbs like palmetto berries, damiana, pumpkin seeds, and foods high in zinc and vitamin E. Exercises designed to strengthen the abdominal and lower back muscles can also be helpful. To stimulate the sexual organs directly, apply Vital Force Contact to the point about one inch below the navel several times a day. These recommendations will *not* increase sexual potency in individuals who already are functioning at their optimal level.

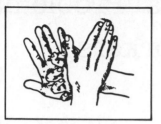

CHAPTER 7

OCCUPATIONAL WEAR AND TEAR:
WHERE YOUR WORK IS HURTING YOU

Most of us spend more time at our work than at any other activity. In this chapter, we have categorized the body problems you may experience as a result of your occupation or the type of work that you do. Specific problems are grouped according to their cause, which can be either direct or indirect. Some occupations may cause imbalances in more than one area. For example, most tailors usually work sitting down. This causes an atrophy of the leg muscles, which may cause the muscles to contract and thus limit flexibility. Tailors also do very close work with their eyes and must always use a good lighting source to reduce strain. Also, this occupation requires the constant use of arms, shoulders, hands, and fingers. After several years some stiffness could develop.

Of course, each individual's body is different. Individual stamina and weaknesses have a great deal to do with the extent of bodily disorder an occupation will cause and the time it takes to correct the disorder, but the fact remains that there are certain imbalances that are common to people who perform certain work activities.

The chart below is a guide to these problems and can be used with the previous chapter, "Body Parts That Hurt," to prevent and correct problems.

Chart 7—1 Occupational Problems: White Collar Workers

BODY PROBLEM	OTHER SYSTEM RECOMMENDED
Atrophy in stomach muscles/ fast food syndrome	Alexander Technique
Back problems	Chiropractic
Cramps in hand/arthritis	Swedish Massage
Eyestrain	Polarity
General muscular atrophy	Exercise
Headaches	T. M. J.
Heart disorders	Shiatsu
Lower back pain	Situps
Mental fatigue	Slant Board (inverted posture)
Pain in wrist & upper arm	Swedish Massage
Shoulder pain	Swedish Massage
Stiff neck	Alexander Technique
Stress overload	Polarity
Throat irritations	Alexander Technique

The day-to-day activities of white collar workers usually demand a great deal of thinking and pondering. Schedules tend to be fast-paced and long hours are spent in meetings, intense conversation, reading, writing, or listening. This can lead to underworked muscles and overweight. The increasing use of microcomputers and word processors in white collar professions have prompted the development of new working skills that increase stress in the shoulders, neck, arms, and eyes. The physical exercise in-

LAWRENCE/HARRISON TECHNIQUE

Technique	Architects	Desk workers/clerks	Executives/Managers	Lawyers	Receptionists	Secretaries/Admin. Assts.	Students	Writers/Editors/Journalists
Gentle Circular Rhythmic Pressure 93	▨	▨	▨	▨	▨	▨	▨	▨
Circular Rhythmic Pressure to Sacrum 73	▨	▨	▨			▨	▨	
Range of Motion to Wrist/Knead Fingers 99	▨		▨					▨
Eye Rotation Exercise 120	▨							▨
Kneading 70	▨	▨	▨	▨	▨	▨	▨	▨
Circular Rhythmic Pressure to Neck 73	▨	▨	▨		▨	▨		▨
Water Balancing 179			▨	▨	▨			
Circular Rhythmic Pressure to Sacrum 73			▨	▨	▨	▨		
Law of Similars 64		▨						
Gentle Rhythmic Pressure 99			▨	▨	▨	▨	▨	
Muscle Rock and Kneading 84	▨			▨	▨	▨		▨
Range of Motion 101		▨	▨	▨	▨	▨		
Visualization 217			▨	▨	▨		▨	
Range of Motion 101				▨	▨	▨		

volved in white collar occupations is often snatchy—getting up and sitting down repeatedly, rushing then waiting—or doing tasks which involve intense small motor activity but never any large motor activity. Add the generally sedentary nature of most travel to and from work and the unhealthy design of most office furnishings and air circulation systems, and what appear to be the cushiest of jobs can be among those that most promote poor health.

Chart 7–2 Occupational Problems: Trade Workers

BODY PROBLEM	OTHER SYSTEM RECOMMENDED
Backaches	Chiropractic
Bruises/injuries	Visualization
Burns	Visualization
Eyestrain	Polarity
Finger pain and stiffness	Amma
Knee problems	Shiatsu
Neck and shoulder problems	Alexander Technique
Nervous disorders	Foot Reflexology
Respiratory problems	Polarity
Skin disorders	Steam Room and Exercise
Stomach disorders	Nutrition
Tightness in jaw	T. M. J.
Wrist problem	Swedish

The acumen and exactitude required in trades creates a very distinct kind of bodily wear and tear. Trade workers are frequently engaged in operating vehicles, equipment, and machinery. Precision is an absolute must. Aside from the stress involved in meeting the deadlines inherent in almost any occupation in the trades, trade workers may have to contort their bodies into awkward positions in order to operate machinery, or, in the case of drivers, they may have to remain for hours in one sitting position. They may be exposed to high voltages or harsh weather conditions or have to inhale harsh emissions from the equipment they operate. Jobs in the trades often appear to be among the most

LAWRENCE/HARRISON TECHNIQUE

TECHNIQUE	Artists (studio)	Carpenters	Chefs/cooks	Construction workers	Drivers (cab, bus)/Pilots	Dry cleaners	Electricians	Firefighters	Jewelers	Painters	Photographers	Repairmen	Tailors
Circular Rhythmic Pressure to Sacrum 73		≈		≈	≈			≈	≈	≈		≈	
Water Balancing 179	≈							≈	≈				
Ice Therapy 179			≈		≈	≈							
Eye Rotation Exercise 120	≈	≈											≈
Knead Fingers 99	≈									≈	≈		
Knead Thigh 143							≈						
Muscle Rock and Kneading 84				≈				≈		≈	≈	≈	
Easing Your Mind 215				≈			≈	≈					
General Rhythmic Pressure to Shoulder Blade and Ribs 63	≈								≈				
Nutrition 189									≈				
Nutrition 189			≈		≈								
Yoga Lion 124										≈			
Range of Motion 99													≈

active—their "macho" image in the media has certainly abetted this perception—but in fact, a trades worker might not get very much more healthy muscular exercise from his or her work than a busy white collar manager.

Hence the focus of massage for trade workers should be to balance the body, since trade professions often emphasize muscles on one side of the body more than the other. Attention must be paid to sore, cramping muscles. General fatigue can also be aided by massage, and with proper exercise can reduce, as well as prevent, the chronic discomfort associated with trade work.

Chart 7–3 Occupational Problems: Service Workers

BODY PROBLEM	OTHER SYSTEM RECOMMENDED
Back strain	Chiropractic
Cramps in hand & fingers	Swedish Massage
Eyestrain	Polarity
Foot & leg pains	Amma
Headaches	T. M. J.
Neck	Alexander Technique
Overweight	Exercise
Shoulder pain	Swedish Massage
Sore muscles	Swedish Massage
Stomach problems	Nutrition
Tension/nervousness	Foot Reflexology
Voice & throat problems	Alexander Technique

Service workers are constantly dealing with the public. Often their jobs involve constant talking, standing, and caring for others. Many service workers are in constant motion, though they may not move beyond a radius of a few yards during their entire workday, or they may repeat the same route or beat day after day. They are among the most active workers, but their activity frequently leads to overuse of the limbs—causing

LAWRENCE/HARRISON TECHNIQUE

Technique	Bank Tellers	Flight attendants	Haircutters	Librarians	Massage therapists	Physicians and nurses	Police officers	Postal workers	Sales personnel	Teachers	Telephone operators	Waiters
Circular Rhythmic Pressure to Sacrum 73				X	X			X			X	X
Range of Motion on Wrist/Knead Fingers 99	X		X	X	X					X	X	
Eye Rotation Exercise 120	X				X						X	
Deep Circular Rhythmic Pressure 73	X	X				X		X	X			X
Circular Rhythmic Pressure to Neck 73								X				
Range of Motion 101		X		X						X	X	
Nutrition 189							X	X				
Muscle Rock and Kneading 84	X	X			X	X	X	X	X	X	X	X
Circular Rhythmic Pressure 73								X				
Visualization for Deep Relaxation 217								X	X			
Tension Techniques 215						X						
Breathing Techniques 216								X	X			

shoulder, leg, and foot problems—and underuse of the torso. The soreness associated with their overused limbs makes service workers prime candidates for the healing properties of massage. The massage should focus on preventing circulatory problems and relieving soreness in overused limbs.

Chart 7—4 Occupational Problems: Performers

BODY PROBLEM	OTHER SYSTEM RECOMMENDED
All types of musculoskeletal injuries	Swedish Massage
Backache	Chiropractic
Chest pain	Shiatsu
Cramps in fingers	Swedish Massage
Cramps in legs	Amma
Feet problems	Foot Reflexology
Lung and breathing problems	Polarity
Problems with joints	Osteopathy
Shoulder pain	Swedish Massage
Stomach problems	Nutrition
Tension	Foot Reflexology
Throat problems	Alexander Technique
Tightness in jaw	T. M. J.
Voice problems	Alexander Technique
Wrist problems	Swedish Massage

Piano players, quarterbacks, dancers, and politicians may not appear, at first glance, to have much in common in the way of body problems that can be solved by massage. But the similarities are actually quite profound. All are affected in the hearing center because they are constantly exposed to loud and, in many cases, persistent, percussive sounds. These sounds may even be amplified by the use of speakers. These are also fast-

LAWRENCE/HARRISON TECHNIQUE

	Actors	Athletes	Dancers	Musicians: wind instrument players	Musicians: string & percussion	Politicians	Vocalists	Radio & TV announcers
Law of Similars 64	▨	▨	▨					
Circular Rhythmic Pressure to Sacrum 73		▨	▨		▨			
Rhythmic Pressure to Chest 111	▨			▨				
Range of Motion to Wrist/Knead fingers 99	▨			▨	▨		▨	
Circular Rhythmic Pressure 87			▨					
Rhythmic Pressure to Foot 94			▨					
Rhythmic Pressure around Shoulder Blade & Ribs 63	▨			▨		▨	▨	
Range of Motion 64		▨	▨		▨			
Muscle Rock and Kneading 84		▨	▨					
Visualizations/Deep Relaxation 217		▨	▨					
Easing Your Mind 215	▨	▨	▨		▨	▨	▨	▨
Range of Motion 101	▨	▨		▨		▨	▨	▨
Yoga Lion 124			▨	▨		▨	▨	▨
Breathing Techniques 216	▨		▨	▨		▨	▨	▨
Range of Motion 99		▨	▨		▨			

paced, high stress professions, often involving frenetic schedules, night "performances," long hours on the road, and compulsory social activities. Our full body massage is especially helpful to those in the performing professions, for it relaxes the muscles, generally reduces body tension, and restores balance to the body. The latter is particularly important to performers whose work tends to require active use of one particular part of the body or one particular system. This leads to overuse of that one area and underuse or even atrophy, of others—serious imbalance. Depending on the performer's occupation, serious attention may need to be paid to a particular area. It is important to remember that working that part of the body alone will not solve the problem. Other— nonailing body parts—should not be ignored, no matter how much in need the ailing part may be. We suggest that half of a massage session be spent working the overused body part alone and that the remaining half be spent working the rest of the body.

More than in most occupations, performers are actively using their bodies in their work, but unfortunately the use is not balanced and frequently becomes abuse. A large percentage of our clients are performers, who come for the health as well as the beauty aspects of massage, and we have found that frequent and consistent bodywork can allay the physical damage and tension buildup inherent in the performing occupations.

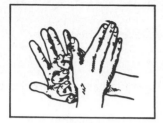

CHAPTER 8

EXERCISE

Exercise has been recognized for centuries as essential for good health. The Greeks, Romans, Egyptians, Indians, and Chinese are just a few of the cultures that followed exercise programs and techniques that were designed to enhance not only physical development, but also moral and emotional development. Massage is actually a form of exercise which is called passive exercise. Regular exercise usually involves self-propelled movement or resistance by the muscles to a fixed point (as in isometrics). In massage there is no self-propelled movement. In massage all movement is carried out by the massage therapist without resistance or assistance of the patient. The ultimate goal remains the same: to increase circulation, range of movement in the joints and greater muscle tone. Massage and exercise go hand in hand. Massage relieves the tightness and soreness that can result from exercise, but proper exercise enhances the effect of massage by improving muscle tone, circulation, and body balancing. Even the best massages, given frequently and consistently, cannot substitute for proper exercise.

With the current concern for total fitness, most of us are now well aware that people need exercise in order to function at their best. However, despite the surge in health club memberships and the hordes of joggers on the streets and in parks, many of us are still not getting enough proper exercise.

To see if you are exercise-deficient, use the following checklist:

_____ tire easily
_____ suffer frequent headaches
_____ back pains
_____ complexion sallow and washed out
_____ overweight
_____ underweight
_____ irritable outbursts

_____ moody and depressed

_____ sleep poorly, have difficulty going to sleep, or wake up tired

_____ difficulty remembering important things

_____ losing interest in sex

_____ body full of tension, aches, and pains that don't seem to have any physical basis

If you checked off five of the above twelve symptoms, you're probably not getting enough exercise or enough of the *right* exercise.

The following exercise program consists of a series of stretching, bending, and aerobic exercises designed to improve muscle tone, increase flexibility in the joints, increase circulation and strengthen the heart, improve mental functioning, bring a glow to the complexion, improve posture, and promote a healthy energy flow.

Altogether, the exercises should take about half an hour a day, and we suggest that they be done in the morning because they will overstimulate you if done at night.

Along with the effects mentioned above, this exercise program will coordinate body and mind and produce greater feelings of calm, serenity, grace, and poise. You will also find most of the exercises fun to do.

Here are some basic rules:

1. Try to exercise at the same time every day.

2. Exercise in a well-ventilated room.

3. Do not eat a heavy meal for an hour before or after doing the exercises; it is likely to cause digestive problems.

4. Wear loose-fitting clothes.

5. For floor exercises use a mat or a folded blanket.

6. Never force your body to do anything.

7. Move through the exercises gradually and slowly; never bend suddenly or bounce into position.

8. After completing each exercise, let your body relax for a few moments.

9. While performing the exercises, focus your mind on specific tensions and blocks and visualize them leaving your body.

10. Pay careful attention to the instructions for breathing and always be careful to breathe deeply and rhythmically.

11. As you gain strength and mastery, gradually increase the difficulty, range of motion, number of repetitions, and fluidity of the exercises.

Breathing

Proper breathing energizes and fortifies the body, aids our thinking processes, increases endurance and stamina, makes us look better, and generally promotes a longer and healthier life. But in spite of the importance of breathing, few of us do it properly. Just as with many natural processes, deep breathing is something that children do automatically but that most adults have forgotten. "Taking a deep breath" sounds like the easiest thing in the world, but for some reason, most people seem almost incapable of doing it with regularity. To some extent this is due to the tension and stresses of our fast-paced life. However, if you want to take advantage of all the wonderful opportunities that life offers, it's definitely to your advantage to learn how to breathe.

There are two basic features to proper breathing: depth and rhythm. Most of us take very shallow breaths, breathing only from the chest or throat. This does not bring enough oxygen into your body, nor does it allow you much control over your voice, which is why singing instructors train their students to breathe from the diaphragm. If you breathe deeply enough, you will almost automatically breathe in the proper rhythm.

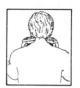

Posture

The way you stand and walk and sit not only can indicate imbalances in different body parts but also can cause problems throughout the body. The entire body works together. Remember that if there is an imbalance in one part, there will be a corresponding imbalance in another. Rounded shoulders can cause headaches and problems in the neck, shoulders, and chest. A protruding pelvis can cause problems in the thighs, legs, and feet. Standing and walking with the weight improperly balanced can contribute to lower back pain. Standing tall and walking proud not only makes you look better and more attractive, it also helps you feel better all over.

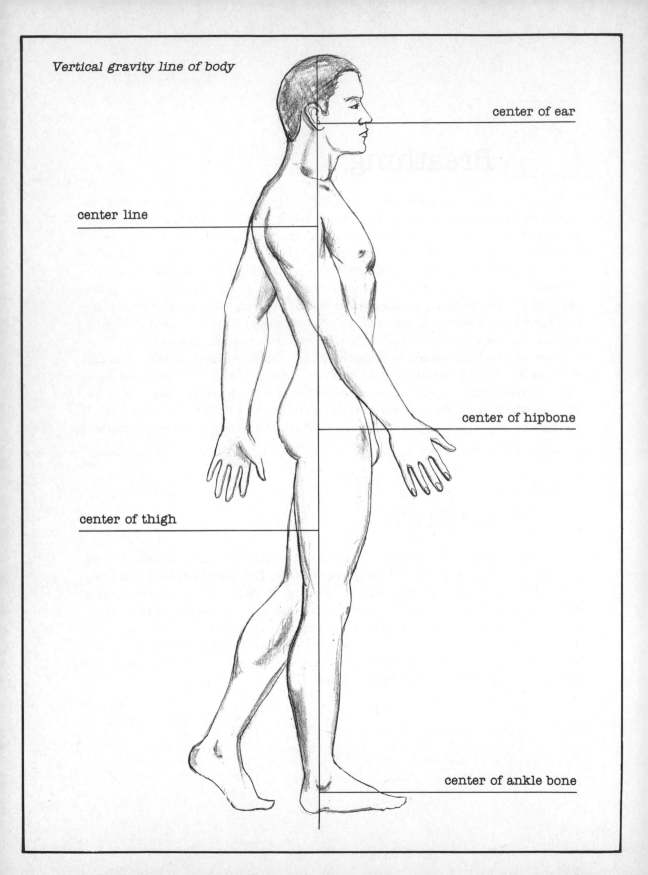

Vertical gravity line of body

center of ear

center line

center of hipbone

center of thigh

center of ankle bone

Daily Exercise Routine

Body Shake

Stand tall. Starting with your feet, shake each part of your body. After shaking your feet, shake your ankles, then the legs, the hips, and the waist, followed by the shoulders, arms and hands, neck, and head.

Purpose: To loosen all the muscles in your body and prepare them for the rest of their exercises; to stimulate the circulation and bring fresh energy to the entire body; to rid the body of tension and negative emotions.

Body Stretch

Stand tall. Raise your arms above your head. Now stretch your arms and fingers as if you were reaching for the stars and clawing the air. As you reach, inhale deeply through your nose while rising onto your toes. Now exhale slowly, and gradually return to your starting position, with your arms hanging loosely at your sides. Repeat this at least three times.

Purpose: to strengthen the Achilles tendon, hamstrings, heart, and shoulders. Also reduces insomnia.

After you have mastered this exercise, increase the difficulty by doing it with your eyes closed.

Body Bend

Stand tall. Slowly bend from the waist, loosely dropping your head and arms. Inhale slowly through your mouth. This will automatically lift your torso. Exhale slowly. This will automatically lower your torso and bring your fingers closer to your toes. Inhale and exhale three times.

> *Caution: If you feel pain behind your knees, bend over only as far as is comfortable or stop the exercise altogether.*

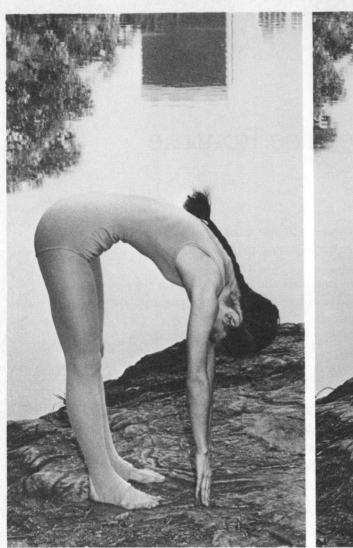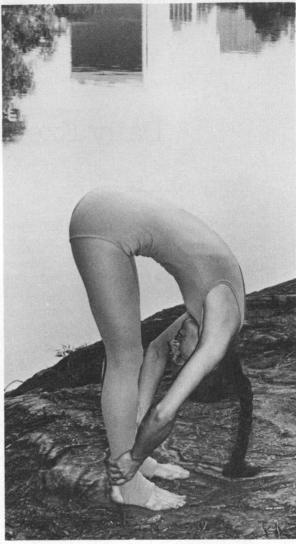

Body bend

Purpose: to stretch hamstrings, back and neck muscles; to tonify and enliven complexion; to relieve congestion in sinuses, nasal passages, and head.

Cradle Stretch

Lie flat on your back. Bend your knees and bring them slowly to your chest, with your arms folded around them. As you are drawing your knees to your chest, inhale deeply.

166

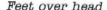

Now exhale, and as you do so draw your legs even closer to your chest. Inhale and exhale three times. Slowly straighten your legs and lower them to the floor.

Purpose: To strengthen lower-back and abdominal muscles.

Leg Lift

Lie flat on your back. Lift your legs off the floor about three feet. Inhale deeply as you are raising your legs. Hold them in this position as long as you can while holding your breath. Then exhale slowly while slowly lowering your legs. Perform three times.

Purpose: strengthens lower back and abdominal muscles and stretches thigh muscles.

After you have mastered this exercise, increase the difficulty by not lifting your legs as high. This will create more tension in your abdominal and back muscles. (See page 133.)

Feet Over Head

Lie flat on your back. Lift your legs off the floor, and try to touch your feet to the floor

Feet over head

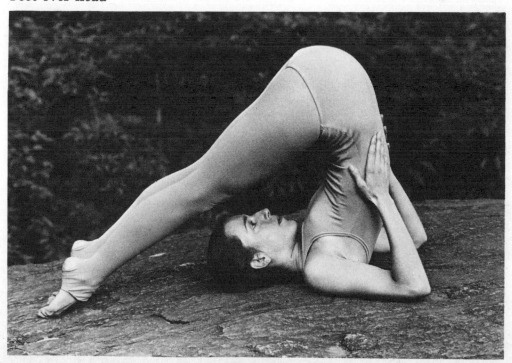

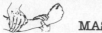

behind your head. If you can't go all the way back, just them take as far as you can. Hold for the count of ten.

Purpose: to tonify entire system and stretch leg, hip, and lower-back muscles.

As the involved muscles begin to stretch and strengthen, you will be able to put your feet farther and farther back.

Cobra

Lie on your stomach. Bend your elbows and place your hands at the sides of your chest. Now raise your chest and feet at the same time. Hold for the count of ten. Slowly lower your body. Repeat three times.

Purpose: to tonify internal organs, stimulate blood flow, and strengthen buttocks and chest muscles. (See page 135.)

Indian-Style Sit

Sit on the floor with your back straight. Cross your legs at the ankles and try to place knees flat on the floor. Don't be discouraged if you can't lay them flat at once. With

Indian-style sit

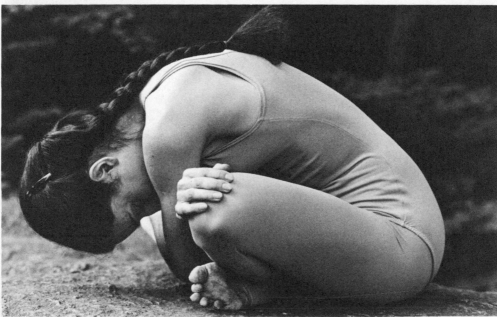

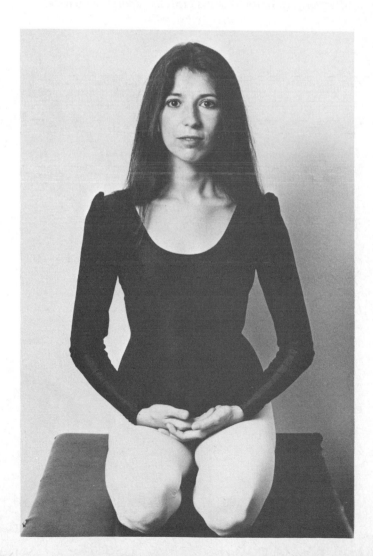

daily practice you soon will be able to. Now cross your arms and place your hands on the opposite knees. While in this position slowly bend from the waist and lower your head as close to the floor as you can. Hold for the count of five.

Purpose: to strengthen the colon, liver, and heart and aid digestion.

Japanese-Style Sit

Kneel on the floor with your legs tucked under you. Try to sit on the floor between your heels. If you can't, then start by sitting on your heels. Now slowly begin to lean back, first resting your hands, then your wrists, then your elbows, then your shoulders

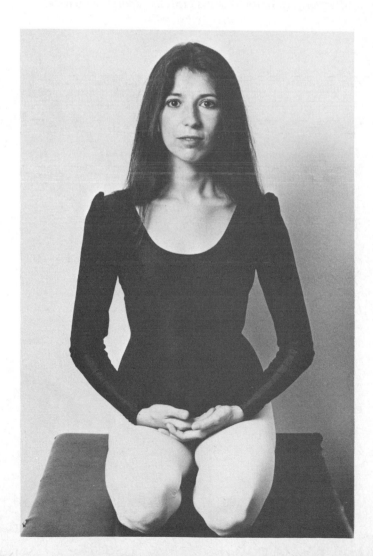

Japanese-style sit

on the floor, ending with your arms straight at your sides. Stop at whatever point you begin to feel discomfort and hold for the count of ten. Slowly return to the starting position.

Purpose: to strengthen pelvic area and abdominal muscles and generally improve sexual functioning.

Riding a Horse

Stand tall, feet together. Now move your right foot to the right about two feet. Point your toes outward at about a 45-degree angle. Holding your back very straight, bend your knees as deep as you can. Hold for the count of five.

Purpose: strengthens shins, thighs, and abdomen.

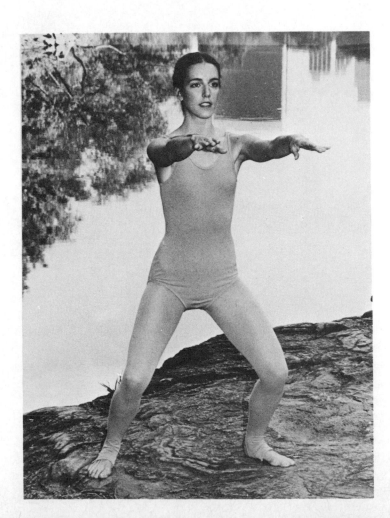

Riding a horse

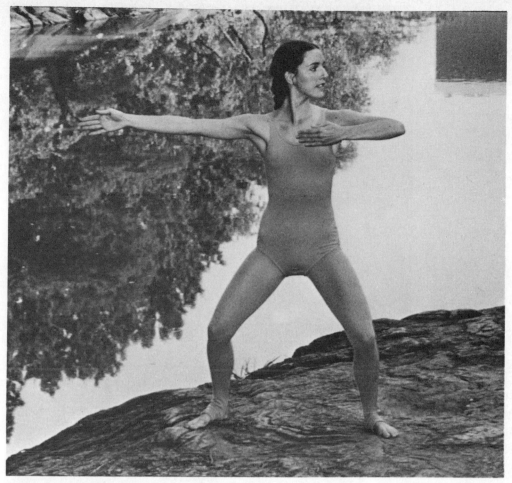

Pulling the bow

Pulling the Bow

Get into the Riding a Horse position. Raise your arms slowly above your knees. Now, as if to pull a bow, extend your right arm across your body, with your right fingers open and spread, and your left hand in a fist. With your left hand stable on the bow, slowly pull your right hand back as if pulling the string, clenching your fist as you go. As you pull your right arm back behind your right shoulder, turn your head to the right, ending with your right arm stretched behind you. Slowly lower your arms. Then raise them again and do the exercise in the opposite direction.

Purpose: to strengthen fingers, arms, shoulders, upper back, and neck.

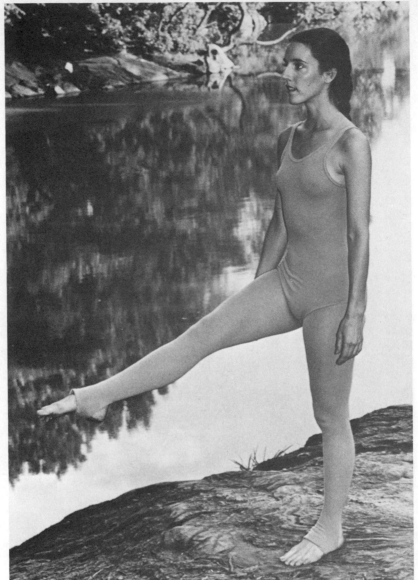

Foot Rotation

Stand tall. Lift one foot about twelve inches from the floor. Flex the foot up and down, six times in each direction. Rotate the foot, twelve times clockwise and twelve times counterclockwise. Repeat for the other foot.

Purpose: to strengthen the toe, foot, and ankle muscles.

172

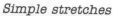

Aerobics

Run in place to a count of 200, gradually increasing to 500
   or
Dance vigorously for at least five minutes to your favorite up-tempo record, being as creative as you can, engaging your whole body, and constantly moving.
Purpose: to stimulate circulation and energize the total system.
Now stretch whatever part of your body feels stiff or knotty. Be creative.

Simple stretches

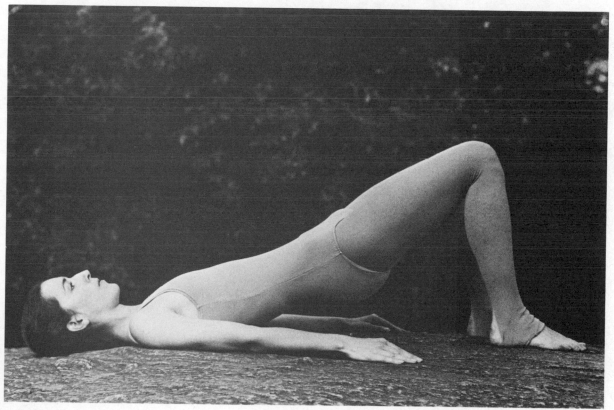

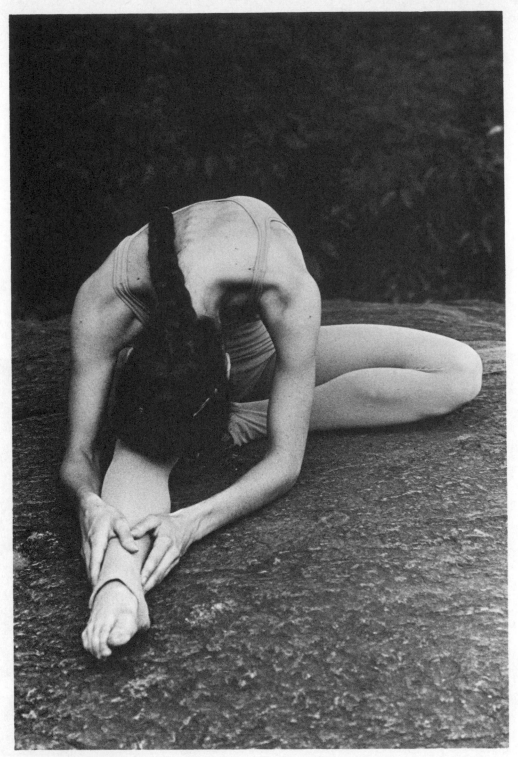

Simple stretches

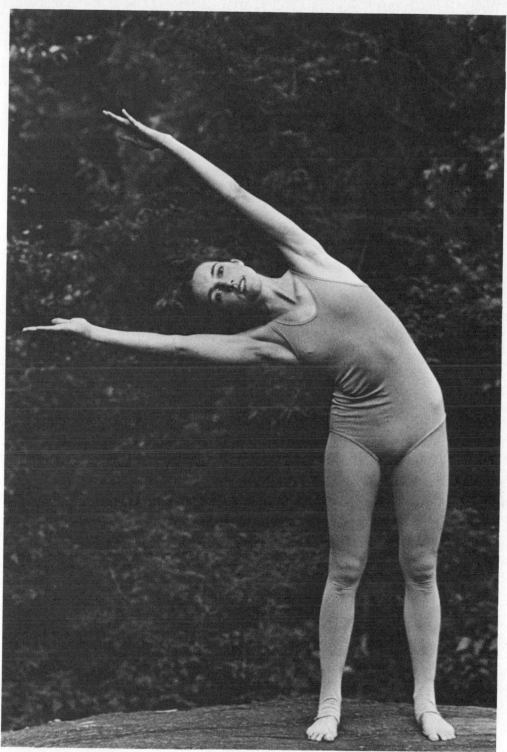

Simple stretches

Gravity Reversal

Do a shoulder stand for five minutes. Gravity reversal techniques help to stretch the spine and increase blood flow to the head and upper extremities. The result of this is reduced stress and a greater sense of health and well being.

Purpose: to clear the mind, stimulate internal organs, purify the blood. Good for thyroid, digestion, nervousness, sinuses, sexual strength, hair, and eyesight.

Putting It All Together

Lie flat on your back and close your eyes. Visualize a natural sea or a landscape that makes you feel very good and experience the energy flowing through your body. Then just rest for a few minutes until you feel like stirring.

Purpose: to induce a feeling of peace, harmony, and tranquility.

Now you can begin your day with the feeling that you are able to do whatever it is that needs to be done.

A Note About Health Clubs

With more and more people taking a greater interest in their physical well-being, health clubs, gymnasiums, and body-building programs are gaining widespread popularity. For many people in our mobile society, they provide an excellent opportunity for social contact. And there are other people—the body builders and the "iron pumpers"—who use clubs to develop their musculature. Most people, however, see them as a convenient and convivial way to stay in good condition. If you are thinking about joining a health club, consider the following:

1. Is it safe, clean, and well staffed with knowledgeable people?
2. Does it have a nurse or a physician available at all times?
3. Does it have adequate equipment and facilities for your needs (e.g., large enough pool, sauna, steam room, whirlpool, exercise classes, Nautilus machines, vapor room)? Consider carefully what your needs are. There is no reason to pay for a full range of facilities when you plan to use only one or two.
4. What is the cost?
5. Is it conveniently located? Is it near your home or your job? If you don't use the

facility regularly because it's not easy to get to, the membership fee will be a waste of money.

6. Does it have branches in other cities? This can be a tremendous asset if you travel a lot. It provides an opportunity to keep up your health program and meet people at the same time.

7. Does the club have a massage therapist on the premises?

Clearly, any program should be tailored to your specific needs and condition. However, the following is a well-rounded, brief health club program that would prove generally beneficial for most people. It takes about an hour and should be done about three times a week.

1. Warm-up stretching exercises
2. Bicycling or jogging (at least one mile)
3. Nautilus exercises. The Nautilus program is a series of movements designed to tone and strengthen muscles throughout the body. Before embarking on a Nautilus program, consult with a knowledgeable instructor who can help you adapt the program to your specific needs. If you have a physical condition that does not allow you to use the machines, do more stretching exercises.
4. Warm shower
5. Pool (swimming is a *total* exercise)
6. Whirlpool
7. Sauna
8. Shower
9. Steam
10. Shower

Some Final Guidelines

Have a physical checkup before you begin a new exercise program. Let your physician know what you are planning to do and find out if you have any health conditions that impose limitations. If you are using a health club, make certain that your instructor knows your medical history and present physical condition. (Many health clubs will want a statement from your physician.)

Know why you are exercising and what you hope to achieve. Some people are primarily interested in cardiovascular fitness; others are concerned with relaxation and freeing themselves of tension; still others are primarily interested in developing muscles. The key is to have a program tailor-made for your needs. This will lead to more immediate results, which will in turn motivate you to continue.

Be consistent. It is better, for example, to run one mile each day than to run seven miles one day and none at all on the remaining six. Not only does consistency bring the best results, but erratic exercise habits often lead to excesses that can cause damage to muscles, bones, connective tissues, and internal organs.

Be persistent. If you don't see results immediately you may get discouraged. Or if you begin to feel better you may think you don't need to continue. In either case, don't stop exercising. If your program doesn't seem to be working, is beginning to bore you, or you seem to be rapidly achieving your goals, vary your routine, add new exercises, or set new goals for yourself. Remember, exercise, to be effective, must be regular and ongoing.

Get the proper equipment for your particular program (exercise mats, sweat suits, weights). There is no need to spend large sums of money. Very often you can make use of things you already have. You can put a couple of blankets or an old comforter on the floor to serve as a pad. You can use 16-ounce cans of food for weights. Any old T-shirt and pair of slacks that do not bind at the waist can serve as an exercise suit.

Make your exercise program convenient. Since it is not necessary to do certain types of exercise every day, especially weight lifting and other strenuous exercises, choose days and times that you know are conducive to keeping your "appointments with your body."

Make your exercise time enjoyable. Choose exercises that you really like to do. Play soft music, burn incense, use soft lights or bright lights, wear your favorite color, use your favorite room. In other words, create an environment that makes you feel good.

Though most people will readily acknowledge the importance of exercise few people give it the same importance as sleep or eating. This is probably due to the fact that we automatically experience ill health when deprived of these while the effects of exercise deprivation—while as dangerous if not more dangerous over the long run as poor dietary and sleep habits—are not experienced immediately. Exercise is essential for good health and for the reduction of stress.

To feel truly healthy, begin a daily exercise program with a weekly massage!

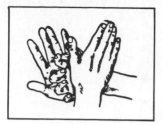

CHAPTER 9

WATER BALANCING

Water balancing is the use of water to prevent or correct imbalances and to improve general well-being. Water balancing helps maintain good health by improving circulation and by increasing the waste elimination activity of the skin and the internal organs. Because water balancing techniques are such an excellent way of either sedating or stimulating the entire system, they are very beneficial adjuncts to massage and bodywork and can be used either before or after a session.

What Does Water Do?

Water plays many roles in our lives. It is essential for life and is a potent therapeutic agent. Human beings can live much longer without food than they can without water. And not drinking enough water can contribute to many physical problems such as dry skin, poor digestion and dehydration. Water distributes nutrients to all the cells of the body, carries wastes out, and comprises two thirds of the body's tissues. For therapeutic effects as an adjunct to massage, water can be used hot or cold, and as a liquid, a solid (ice), or a gas (steam). When combined with herbs and other agents, its therapeutic effects are often enhanced. With massage or bodywork, water helps to loosen and relax muscles.

The water balancing techniques described in this chapter can be used to:

○ Relieve muscle pain due to cramps and spasms.
○ Relax tight muscles.

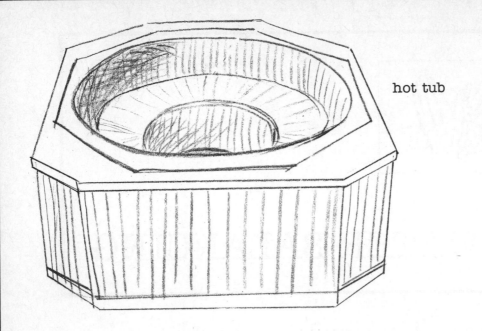

hot tub

whirlpool

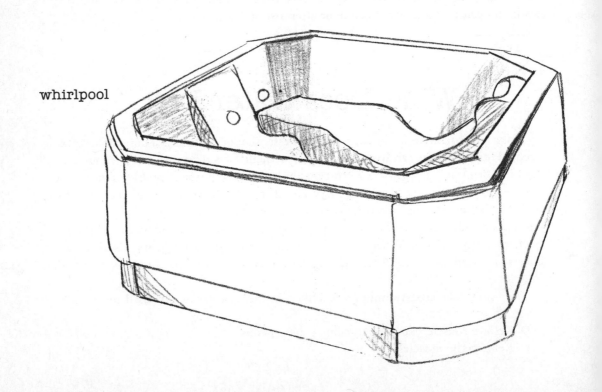

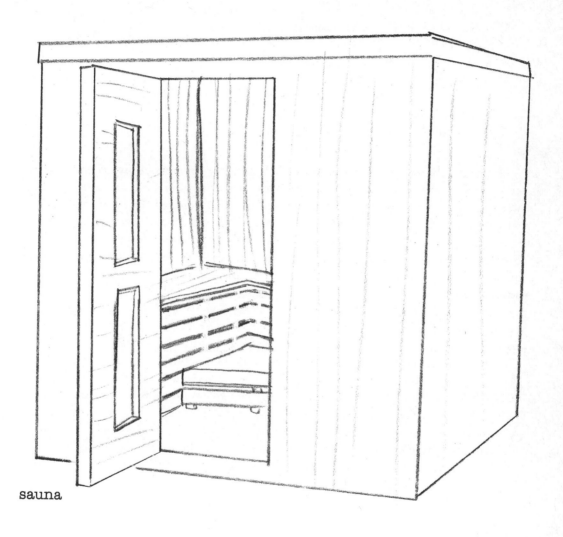

sauna

Ultra-modern water treatments

○ Develop muscle tone.
○ Reduce inflammation.
○ Stimulate sluggish circulation.
○ Reduce swelling.
○ Raise or lower body temperature.
○ Stop bleeding.
○ Purify the body by removing wastes.
○ Relieve constipation.
○ Relieve congestion of blood, lymph, and other body fluids.
○ Unclog the skin.
○ Stimulate or sedate the nervous system.

Water has been used as an integral part of health care throughout history and in many cultures. Sanskrit writings as early as 4000 B.C. report healing baths and other kinds of water therapy, or hydrotherapy. Descriptions of water cures are found in old Tibetan writings. The Babylonians, Egyptians, Cretans and Persians used water therapy extensively, long before the Romans left luxurious baths all over Europe. The Spartans immersed newborn babies in ice-cold water to toughen them and to immunize them against disease. Galen, a Greek physician of the second century A.D., was a firm advocate of the baths that were so popular in Rome and used them with massage and exercise to effect his cures. In the fifteenth century, the Turks popularized the hot-air bath, which is still popularly referred to as the "Turkish bath." American Indians used baths to cure many diseases and had developed vapor baths into a high art.

In the early part of the nineteenth century, Vincent Priesnitz, an uneducated Austrian farmer's son who had been crippled in an accident, cured himself with water treatments. News of his cure spread, and eventually royalty and government officials came to him for help and the water cure became fashionable in Europe. His efforts were so successful that he eventually won the backing of the Austrian government. In 1876 Dr. John Harvey Kellogg opened his famous sanitarium in Battle Creek, Michigan, where his success did a great deal to establish hydrotherapy as an important scientific system.

How to Use Water

Practically everyone uses water balancing in one form or another as part of a regular health-care program. Soaking tired, aching feet; taking a long, hot shower to wake up in the morning; relaxing in a warm tub at night; or using steam baths, saunas, whirlpools, hot tubs, vaporizers, and room humidifiers—all of these are common and easily available forms of water balancing.

Hot Water or Cold?

Temperature is a very important aspect of water's therapeutic value. As a rule, warm water is used for relaxation, hot water to relieve various types of aches and pains, and cold water for stimulation and to conquer fatigue. The following is a guide to water temperatures (all temperatures referred to in this chapter will be Fahrenheit temperatures):

Cold:	40° to 60°F.
Cool:	60° to 70°F.
Tepid:	70° to 90°F.
Warm:	90° to 100°F.
Hot:	100° to 110°F.

Above 110 degrees, water loses its therapeutic value and actually has a negative effect on the body (unless in the form of steam), causing destruction of tissues, desensitizing of nerves, congestion of body fluids, and reduced blood pressure, which can cause dizziness.

Hot water is recommended for sedating the system, relaxing muscle spasms, and relieving pain due to muscle stiffness or irritation. Hot water should *not* be used:

1. when there is swelling or inflammation. Hot water increases blood flow and can therefore cause inflamed, congested blood vessels to rupture.

2. if you are overtired. Heat lowers blood pressure and can cause dizziness.

3. if you have high or low blood pressure, a heart condition, or diabetes, because of the danger of going into shock.

4. when muscles are flaccid.

Cold water stimulates the system and is effective in reducing swelling, inflammation, and the flow of blood to specific organs or parts. It is also useful for increasing muscle tone. It should not be used:

1. when there are open abrasions.

2. in cases of diabetes, heart problems, or any condition involving poor circulation.

Neither very hot nor very cold water should be used when there is a loss of sensation in the skin due to nerve damage or some other condition. In such a situation, hot water can cause serious burns and cold water can cause frostbite, because you will not feel the extremes of temperature. Using extremely hot or cold water excessively can have the same effect—that is, it can cause the nerve damage that leads to desensitization.

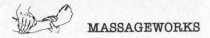

The effects described for hot and cold water apply to most individuals. However, some people react differently. The particular response will depend on climate, the individual's overall health and vitality level, and other personal factors. *If you have any serious medical problems you should first check with your physician before using hot or cold water therapeutically.*

Baths and Showers

Hot Baths

For a hot bath, the temperature should be between 100 and 110 degrees. Anything above this is dangerous, especially for the neophyte.

If you are not accustomed to taking hot baths, gradually condition your body by starting with warm water (about 95 degrees) and slowly increasing the temperature. The goal is to be able to tolerate between 108 and 110 degrees.

A hot bath should last about fifteen minutes. If the water begins to cool, add more hot water to maintain the temperature. Once you have become conditioned to hot baths, you may want to stay in longer. But be warned that if you stay too long, you may emerge looking something like a prune, though this lasts only about fifteen minutes.

Hot baths are valuable for cleansing the skin of bacteria and dead cells, especially when used with a loofah (a type of natural-fiber sponge), a natural-bristle bath brush, or a bath mitt, and getting rid of aches and pains caused by muscle strain or diseases such as arthritis, rheumatism, gout, and neuritis.

To help relieve general stiffness and soreness, put on a terry-cloth robe after taking a hot bath, get into bed, and cover up well with blankets, particularly your head and feet. You probably will perspire for a while and feel somewhat enervated. Stay in bed for several hours. When you get up, dry yourself thoroughly, and gently rub your entire body with a towel dampened with cold water; then dry again slowly. Finish by applying a body-moisturizing oil or lotion.

Certain agents can be put into a hot bath to create helpful effects. One or two cups of Epsom salts in a tub of water is extremely good for relieving aches and pains. Although it is sometimes used as a laxative, we recommend it for external use only. Used externally, it stimulates the eliminatory activity of the skin and glands and rids the body of harmful toxins and waste. This effect can be obtained with ordinary table salt, but to a lesser extent.

Cold Baths

Cold baths should last only about three or four minutes. They are used primarily to stimulate the circulation of blood, thereby invigorating the entire system. They are also helpful in combatting inflammation and swelling.

On first impact, cold water tightens the superficial capillaries, driving the blood to the inner body. Then the superficial capillaries gradually expand and the blood returns to the surface. The circulatiton of blood is aroused and the entire body is energized.

> *Caution:* Because cold water lowers body temperature quickly, do not use for long periods of time.

Lukewarm Baths

Spending twenty minutes stretched out in a tub of lukewarm water can do more to calm your nerves than can any number of tranquilizers. To make your bath a really sensuous and luxurious experience, add an oil that has a sedating effect, such as pine, rose, or jasmine; burn a similar incense; add food coloring to the water to turn it sea blue or lavender; use soft lights and quiet music. Then focus on your senses—the sound of the music, the smell of the oil and incense, the feeling of the water on your body.

Hot and Cold Showers

Showers, whether hot or cold, are more invigorating than baths. The action of the water over the body's surface helps to increase the stimulation. It's for this reason that many people are addicted to showers and can't start the day without them. For these people, a shower is not so much a necessity for getting clean but for waking up.

One of the simplest and most powerful ways to energize yourself is with the alternating hot and cold shower. Not everyone will enjoy or be able to tolerate this technique. But for those who are willing and able to try it, the effects are astonishing.

1. Stand under a hot shower for about three minutes.

2. Slowly increase the cold water while shutting down the hot. Allow the water to become as cold as you can stand it.

3. To avoid shocking your nervous system, run the cold water onto your right foot and leg first, since this is the point farthest from the heart. The spray can then be directed to different parts of the body.

4. Spray with cold water ten to thirty seconds; then turn back to hot.

5. Repeat the sequence three times. The entire shower should take no more than ten minutes.

6. When finished, rub yourself vigorously with a thick terry cloth towel and apply a moisturizing cream or oil.

This technique quickly and dramatically strengthens the body's vital energy, especially when the cold water is directed onto the genitals and the back of the neck. Always start with hot water and end with cold.

> **Caution:** *If you have a heart condition, check with your physician before using this technique.*

Whirlpools, Underwater Massage, Aerated Baths

These baths are excellent invigorating techniques.

In underwater massage, the water is directed to different parts of the body by individual jets. This method, which can come in the form of a bath or a shower, is most likely to be found in a health club or spa, but is occasionally found in older, luxury hotels.

In the whirlpool bath, which is similar to underwater massage, small agitators are used to circulate the water around the body. Although whirlpools are most often found in health clubs and resorts, there are numerous machines on the market that can turn your bathtub into a whirlpool.

Aerated baths involve the use of compressed air to create bubbles that produce a gentle pressure around the body.

Whirlpool baths are commonly used in sports medicine and physical therapy to relax tense and strained muscles. They are also useful in healing fractures and treating paralysis, wounds, and sprains. Aerated baths and underwater massage can also bring relief from these conditions.

Steam Baths

A steam bath followed by a short cold shower is both purifying and invigorating. Steam is excellent for unclogging the pores in the skin and helping the body eliminate harmful toxins and waste material.

Steam is often used to relieve congestion in the sinuses and respiratory tract as well as to cleanse facial pores. The following is a simple way to accomplish both goals at once.

1. Boil four quarts of water. Add three tablespoons of an herbal laxative, and ten drops of eucalyptus oil and steep for five minutes.

2. Place the kettle on a table; sit with your head over it; cover your head and the kettle with a large towel so that all the steam will be directed toward your face.

3. Remain in this position for about fifteen minutes. When you first start using this technique, you may need to come out from under the towel several times until you get accustomed to the heat, or you may want to stay under the towel for only about five minutes.

4. When you have finished, splash your face with cold water and apply a moisturizing cream.

Foot Baths

Soaking your feet is a very popular and effective water balancing technique.

The most effective treatment for tired and aching feet is to alternate baths of hot and cold water, which should at least cover your ankles and, preferably, reach an inch or two above them. Start with hot water and soak for three to five minutes. Then put your feet in cold water for half a minute to a minute. Repeat this sequence three times, *ending with cold water*. When you are finished, dry your feet vigorously.

If you do not feel you can take the alternating hot and cold water, soak your feet in hot water with Epsom salts for about twenty minutes, adding hot water when necessary to maintain the temperature. Dry briskly when finished.

Which ever type of foot bath you use, the most refreshing way to finish is to apply firm General or Circular Rhythmic Pressure to the soles of your feet, rub on a light body oil or cream, and then apply cornstarch. This is guaranteed to leave you feeling refreshed all over.

Another relaxing and energizing water-balancing technique for the feet, and the entire body, is to walk barefoot in dewy grass or wet sand for fifteen minutes to a half hour. These surfaces make excellent conductors of energy from the earth into the body. Finish by drying and massaging your feet thoroughly and then taking a brisk walk in dry socks and shoes.

Sitz Baths

The *sitz bath,* which can be taken either hot or cold or by alternating the two, is used to treat abdominal, genital, and rectal problems. One of the most common uses in the home is for relief of hemorrhoid discomfort and chronic constipation.

In the *sitz bath,* only the hip area is immersed in water. Health establishments use a tub that is divided into two sections, one filled with cold water, the other with hot. This enables the patient to take alternating hot and cold baths.

When taking a *sitz bath* at home, sit in about four inches of water if you are taking a hot sitz bath and about ten inches if you are taking a cold one. Keep your feet out of the water by resting them against the end of the tub. You can use a towel under your feet to keep them from sliding. A cold *sitz bath* should last only two or three minutes and definitely no longer than five. A hot sitz bath, with the temperature about 108 degrees, should last about five minutes, or until the water approaches body temperature.

Cold *sitz baths* are excellent for stimulating the energy flow in the pelvis and lower abdomen and tonifying the nerves in this area. They are also helpful for chronic constipation. They are, however, contraindicated when there is inflammation or pus in any part of this area. Hot *sitz baths* are recommended for reducing nervous tension.

Alternating hot and cold *sitz baths* are recommended for strained hip muscles, muscle spasms in the lower back, hemorrhoids, and general toning. They can be taken at home by using the bathtub for hot water and a large metal tub for cold water from the tap. The hot water should be kept at a temperature around 104 degrees. Start with hot water and soak for about two minutes; then soak about one minute in the cold water. Alternate four times, always ending with the cold water.

> *Caution:* Women should not take sitz baths immediately before, during, or after the menstrual period. (Sitz baths may cause abdominal congestion, which could lead to cramps.)

Compresses and Packs

Compresses and packs are a convenient way to apply the healing properties of water to specific body parts. They are, in general, used for the same purposes as baths and showers. The method to choose will depend on the specific body part and problem.

A compress is a piece of fabric several inches wide (the exact size depends on the body part) and long enough to wrap around the part in question with some overlap so that it can be secured with a safety pin. Compresses are best made out of linen or a linenlike fabric and then wrapped in wool flannel. To apply moist heat to an area, first soak a piece of linen or muslin of the proper size in *cold* water, wring out the water, and apply the compress. Now wrap this in warm wool flannel. Within about ten minutes, the compress should be warm. Compresses should be kept on for several hours or overnight.

The waist compress is a multi-purpose treatment that can aid in the absorption of nutrients, relieve constipation, improve circulation, reduce fevers, and help get rid of headaches. Use fabric eight inches wide and long enough to encircle the waist. After the material has been soaked in cold water and wrung out, wrap it around the waist and then cover it with several layers of wool flannel. The heat from your body will warm the compress in about fifteen minutes. It should be applied before retiring and left on overnight.

Packs are made of several layers of flannel cut to the appropriate size and placed on the afflicted area. They are used locally to treat injuries or inflammation. First, soak the pack in very hot water than wring it out and apply to the afflicted area, leaving it on for only two or three minutes. Then replace it with a cold pack soaked in tap water, letting it remain for only one minute. Repeat the sequence for ten to twenty minutes, depending on the severity of the problem and the condition of the patient. The pack should always cover the area completely.

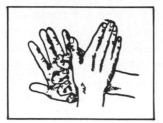

CHAPTER 10

NUTRITION

Nutrition is often either oversimplified or overcomplicated. Our intention is to help clear up some of the confusion.

The nutrients—vitamins, proteins, carbohydrates, fats, and minerals—plus sunlight, air, and water play an essential role in the maintenance of the human body. Proteins, vitamins, minerals, and water build up and heal the body. Carbohydrates, fats, and proteins energize it.

Disorders such as excessive fatigue, poor circulation, and deterioration of muscle, bones, and vital organs can be improved by massage, but if you pay careful attention to what you eat, unnecessary health problems can often be prevented. The more active you are, the more vulnerable you will be to musculoskeletal imbalances that result in injuries to bones, muscles, tendons, and ligaments, therefore, a healthy diet is essential if you lead a busy, fast-paced life.

An excuse that many people give for poor eating habits is that nutrition is a controversial area, with new and contradictory theories arising every day. This is true to some extent. But at the same time, there are a vast number of nutritional concepts based on sound research that have broad general acceptance.

The purpose of this chapter is to give you a good, commonsense understanding of basic nutrition and a clear guide to making intelligent choices.

> **Note:** *Various health problems may be due to allergic reactions to foods. Food allergies may mimic hundreds of other health problems. These may include digestive difficulties, headaches, shortness of breath, mental confusion, and dizziness. If you are experiencing a reaction that you think might be due to a food allergy, check with a qualified nutritional consultant or an allergist.*

Nutrition is a vital living process that involves not only eating and digestion of food but thousands of other processes. The blood carries nutrients to the various cells and tissues throughout the body, feeding the muscles and nerves and thus restoring vital force, so your body can function optimally. Massage, by the effect it has on stimulating circulation, has an important role in bringing nutrients to the cells. People under constant stress will experience greater emotional problems than will the rest of the population. Such exaggerated stress may result in ulcers, colitis, and poor absorption of nutrients, even from the most well-balanced diets. Massage has the ability to reduce this stress and tension and thereby increase the body's ability to absorb nutrients and use them more efficiently. So massage improves the quality of your nutrition.

Although most nutritionists suggest following Recommended Daily Allowances for certain nutrients, the fact remains that different people have different nutritional requirements. Food needs are determined by a person's gender, age, life style and stress as well as emotional factors. Thus a weight lifter will require greater amounts of protein for the building of muscle and a long-distance runner will require greater amounts of unrefined complex carbohydrates for energy to burn on the track. Office workers may require foods high in vitamin C and the B complex because of the high stress level of their jobs; beans, grains, and fresh vegetables are a good choice. Construction workers, on the other hand, burn lots of energy and use lots of muscle; thus, fresh fruits along with nuts and seeds are indicated.

Good, balanced nutritional habits help you to function under the stress that you experience every day. Living in these unpredictable and rapidly changing times has left most of us physically and mentally unprepared to defend against the stress of water, air, and noise pollution as well as the many subtle stresses we come in contact with every day. It doesn't matter if the stress is physical or psychological, the body responds to it in the same way. Whether you injure yourself or argue with your mate or best friend, run from a charging elephant or eat too much sugar, the body responds the same way—the only difference being in degree. Regular massage as well as a good diet will help you to maintain an emotional and a physical balance.

Remember that as important as nutrition and massage are, they are only two factors in your quest for reduced stress and optimum fitness. In order to experience true health, you must practice a total approach: proper diet, exercise of a noncompetitive nature, and a positive attitude, in addition to massage. Only when all these factors are balanced, can you hope to eliminate the effects of tension and stress upon your body and realize the benefits of true good health.

Whatever your eating habits, they probably can stand improvement, and you can get more nutrition from your food dollar. Changing eating habits is not easy, but with motivation, knowledge, and a little self-discipline, it can be done.

Motivation. First, you must seriously want to change your eating habits. You must also be very clear about why you want to change and what you hope to achieve. You must be assured that better nutrition can help you solve your health-related problems, have more energy, eliminate unnecessary aches and pains, deal more effectively with stress, retard the aging process, and generally live a healthier and more fulfilling life.

Knowledge. The more you know about nutrition, the more likely you are to make sound decisions. Sophistication in this area has grown rapidly in recent years, and there are many good books and magazines that can help you expand your knowledge.

Self-discipline. In the final analysis, determination and will power will be the deciding factors. You can't eat whole, nutritious food today and empty, junk foods tomorrow and hope to be nutritionally sound. You must eat nutritious foods on a regular basis if they are to help you improve and maintain your health.

The Essential Nutrients

The major nutrient groups are proteins, carbohydrates, fats, vitamins, minerals, and water. They are responsible for the following functions:

Proteins

- Growth and repair of body tissues.
- Structure of body cells.
- Maintenance of normal fluid balance.
- Regulation of body functions.
- Production of antibodies to fight infection and disease.

Carbohydrates

- Main source of energy for all tissues, including the brain and nervous system.
- Source of glucose for nerve tissues.

Fats

- Concentrated source of energy.

○ Source of essential fatty acids.
○ Transportation and absorption by body cells of fat-soluble vitamins A,
　D, E, and K.

Vitamins

○ Maintenance of body processes.
○ Effective use of other nutrients.
○ Normal physical and mental development.

Minerals

○ Building materials for bones, teeth, and other tissues such as blood and
　nerves.
○ Regulation of body processes.
○ Maintenance of normal fluid and acid/base balance.

Water

○ Essential, major constituents of all body cells.
○ Removal of waste from the body.

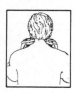

Protein and Its Sources

The finest protein elements are those derived from vegetables. Although some varieties of vegetable protein are not utilized as efficiently as animal protein, many vegetable proteins are utilized more efficiently. Poultry, meat, fish, and eggs have many good nutritional qualities; however, because of present farming and food production techniques, especially the use of pesticides and other chemicals, as well as the cruelty involved in factory farming, their value as primary sources of nutrition should be seriously questioned.

The following is a list of the best sources of vegetable proteins:

○ Sunflower seeds or meal, raw and unsalted.

- ○ Hulled sesame seeds or meal.
- ○ Raw nuts such as almonds, pine nuts (pignolias), Brazil nuts, and pecans. Ground meal or butters of these nuts are also excellent, but should always be made of raw and unsalted nuts.
- ○ Soy beans and garbanzo beans (chickpeas). These should be soaked overnight so that they will not require much cooking. Dried lentils, kidney beans, lima beans, and split peas are also fine protein foods. Beans form an even higher quality protein when combined with sesame seeds or grains such as rice, millet, or corn.
- ○ Brewer's and nutritional yeasts are the source of the finest vegetable proteins. We recommend brands that are calcium-magnesium balanced.
- ○ Bee pollen pellets are a fine source of protein as well as of B vitamins.
- ○ Raw milk products and high quality dairy foods are fine protein sources unless you are allergic. Certified dairy products are safest and healthiest.
- ○ Tofu (bean curd).
- ○ Tempeh (a natural replacement for many meat products).
- ○ Micro algae, usually available in table or powder form, are also a good source of B_{12}. Two popular varieties are spirulina and chlorella.

Vitamins and Their Sources

Vitamins are essential body-building elements and play an important role in the prevention of illness. Fresh fruits and vegetables are the best sources of these nutrients, which are destroyed when food is overexposed to air, heat, and light.

Vitamins	Best Sources	Functions
Vitamin A	fish, cabbage, carrots, celery, dandelions, spinach, watercress, oranges	Aids skin, eyes, liver, bone growth, kidney, muscles, lungs, and heart function.
Thiamine (B_1)	brewer's yeast, whole grains, wheat germ	Helps build and nurture cells. Breaks down carbohydrates.
Riboflavin (B_2)	brewer's yeast, whole grains, wheat germ	Helps carry hydrogen and oxygen through the body.
Niacin (B_3)	brewer's yeast, whole grains, wheat germ	Affects the skin, nerves, digestion, and vision.

Vitamins	Best Sources	Functions
Pyridoxine (B$_6$)	brewer's yeast, whole grains, wheat germ, potatoes, green, leafy vegetables	Helps build blood cells and control cholesterol, which in excessive amounts can cause a blockage in blood flow and lead to hardening of the arteries.
Vitamin B$_{12}$	Many nutrition books claim that animal proteins are the only sources for this vitamin; however, large amounts can be obtained from micro-algae like spirulina and chlorella as well as from dairy products	Essential for normal functioning of all cells, particularly bone marrow, the nervous system, and the digestive system. Needed for red blood cell formation.
Biotin	brewer's yeast, wheat germ	Essential in the formation of nucleic acid and glycogen. Is required in the synthesis of several of the nonessential amino acids, which are building blocks of protein.
Pantothenic Acid	tomatoes, nuts, potatoes, green vegetables, and molasses	Helps to maintain blood sugar and to resist body stress.
Folic Acid	green, leafy vegetables, brewer's yeast	Sparks action from vitamins A, D, E, and K. Also affects the liver, kidneys, and blood.
Vitamin C	lemons, oranges, grapefruit, green peppers, tomatoes, berries, rose hips, watercress	Helps form red blood cells, protects and promotes bone and tissue growth, and builds the body's resistance to disease. Acts as a catalyst to spark action of other vitamins.
Vitamin D	cod liver oil	Helps preserve calcium and phosphorus in the blood. Nourishes the blood.
Vitamin E	green, leafy vegetables, wheat germ, vegetable oils, nuts, whole grains	Breaks up cholesterol. Is a healing agent. Increases stamina.
Vitamin F	pumpkin seeds, sunflower seeds, other nuts	Keeps tissues functioning.
Vitamin K	watercress, cabbage and other green vegetables	Helps clotting of blood.

Minerals and Their Sources

Minerals are the essential building materials of the body and were recognized as essential to human nutrition long before vitamins were discovered. Although vitamins are used by the body in relatively small amounts, many minerals are needed in quantities of one gram or more. Minerals are more important in our diets than many people realize, and most diets are seriously deficient in them. Neither muscles nor nerves can function properly unless they are bathed in tissue fluids that contain certain amounts of mineral salts.

Minerals	*Best Sources*	*Functions*
Calcium	dairy products, dark-green vegetables, nuts, beans, and seeds	Develops bones and teeth. Assists in the movement of muscles and the clotting of blood.
Chloride	kelp and other sea vegetables	Though seldom discussed, is part of hydrochloric acid, which is used in digestion. Also affects muscle functioning and provides life-sustaining elements.
Chromium	brewer's yeast	Increases the effectiveness of insulin and stimulates the enzyme involved in glucose metabolism.
Cobalt	soy beans	Essential for the formation of vitamin B_{12}.
Copper	green, leafy vegetables	An essential mineral found in all body tissues, though very little is required.
Iodine	kelp, sea vegetables, turnip tops	Was first nutrient considered essential to human beings. Affects the thyroid gland and many metabolic functions of the body.

Minerals	Best Sources	Functions
Iron	molasses, green, leafy vegetables, sea vegetables, raisins, apricots	Provides oxygen and helps it to be utilized by the body.
Magnesium	soy flour, whole wheat, brown rice, nuts, beans, molasses	Stimulates brain impulses and muscle contractions. Affects the glands.
Manganese	bananas, beans, wheat bran, celery, nuts	Is an important catalyst and component of many enzymes in the body.
Phosphorus	beans, soy flour, whole wheat	Has more functions than any other mineral, including the formation of strong bones and teeth.
Potassium	bananas, oranges, green, leafy vegetables, nuts, beans	Stimulates nerve impulses for muscle contraction. Helps maintain water balance and distribution. Necessary for healthy functioning of the adrenal glands.
Selenium	brewer's yeast	Serves as an anti-oxidant and is believed to be a cancer prevention agent.
Sodium	celery, kelp, and other sea vegetables	Works with chloride to regulate the pH balance of body fluids.
Sulfur	wheat germ, beans, cheese, peanuts, garlic	Maintains sugar level in the blood. Affects the hair and all cells.
Zinc	pumpkin seeds, beans (especially lentils), peas, spinach	Is a component of insulin. Stimulates the enzymes involved in digestion and metabolism.

Additional minerals that have a place in nutrition are vanadium, molybdenum, nickel, tin, silicon, aluminum. Minerals that have no known requirement and can be toxic include cadmium, lead, and mercury.

Carbohydrates and Their Sources

Carbohydrates are a primary source of energy and a major source of bulk or fiber. There are many types of carbohydrates, and they are generally classified by their molecular complexity. For example, there are many sugars: simple monosaccharides (which include glucose, fructose, and galactose); disaccharides (which include sucrose, maltose, and lactose); and polysaccharides (which include starch, destrines, cellulose, and glycogen). *(For definitions, see glossary.)*

Healthy diets should contain a predominance of unrefined, complex carbohydrates. These are whole grains like wheat, millet, brown rice, and buckwheat groats; roots and rootlike vegetables such as potatoes and carrots; and legumes (beans). Simpler carbohydrates containing glucose, fructose, and galactose may be used in moderation. The best sources for these are fresh fruits.

Green, leafy vegetables are a good source of cellulose, which is a nondigestible carbohydrate and a source of the fiber and bulk that is necessary for stimulating and cleansing the gastrointestinal tract and for proper bowel movements.

In addition to providing energy for the body and bulk for the diet, carbohydrates have the following functions:

1. If there are not enough carbohydrates present, the body will be forced to use protein as an energy source.

2. Carbohydrates contribute to the metabolism of fats, making them available for physical energy. Insufficient intake of carbohydrates results in excessive amounts of fats being used for energy.

3. Carbohydrates help to detoxify the body by converting certain chemicals, bacterial toxins, and some normal metabolites into a form that can be excreted as waste.

4. Certain carbohydrate foods—beans, brown rice, wheat—supply significant quantities of protein, minerals, and B vitamins.

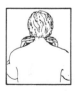

Fats and Their Sources

Fat is an oily yellow or white substance that is formed in animals and vegetables. Its main function in the body is to provide a concentrated form of energy.

Fats are composed of units known as fatty acids, some of which have special properties that make them solid at room temperature. These are known as saturated fatty acids. Fatty acids that are liquid at room temperature (usually called "oils") are generally known as unsaturated fatty acids. Most animal fats are saturated; most fats from vegetable origins are unsaturated, with the exception of avocado, coconut, and other palm fats.

There is much research available that indicates that diets high in saturated fats can lead to many health problems, including heart disease. Some vegetable oils are made saturated by a chemical process known as hydrogenation, the process that is used to manufacture margarine and vegetable shortening. Though these products contain no cholesterol, about which there is a great deal of controversy, they are nevertheless difficult to digest.

The three fatty acids that are essential to the body are linoleic acid, linolenic acid, and arachidonic acid. These fatty acids are like vitamins and minerals in that they must be obtained from food sources because the body cannot manufacture them. A deficiency in these fatty acids can lead to imbalances ranging from something as simple as dry skin to serious neuromuscular disorders.

The best and most desirable sources for the three essential fatty acids are vegetables, nuts, and seeds. Sunflower seeds, pumpkin seeds, and almonds are particularly rich in this nutrient.

Fat in the diet serves the following functions:

- It provides a concentrated form of vitamin E and is the form in which this vitamin is stored in the body.
- It makes it possible for the body to use proteins in the diet to manufacture tissue.
- It creates a cushioning effect for internal organs and tissues and helps to hold them in place.
- It conserves body heat and helps maintain body temperature.
- It helps to transport and absorb the fat-soluble vitamins A, E, D, and K.
- It slows down the emptying time of the stomach, and provides a feeling of fullness and satisfaction.
- It adds to the flavor of food.

Supplementation

As a result of the mounting stresses of modern life and the increased concern about physical fitness, many people are now taking vitamin and mineral supplements. Owing to the devitalization of many of our foods—the loss of nutrients through overcooking, improper storage, and poor farming practices—vitamin and mineral supplementation can be of value in many situations. However, care must be taken when planning a nutrition program, since further nutritional imbalances can be created if excessive amounts of supplementation are used. This is especially true in the improper use of mineral supplements. To produce good results, supplementation programs must be tailored to individual needs, based on gender, age, level of activity, eating patterns, and other factors such as environment, occupation, and medical history.

If you are seriously considering a supplementation program, it would be wise to visit a qualified nutritional consultant who can help you plan a program based on your personal needs.

Rules for Healthy Eating

Here are a few general guidelines on which to base a healthy diet.

1. *Do not overeat.* Do not eat the meal of a boxer when you do the work of a secretary. Foods that are not utilized after they are eaten become part of the waste inside your body. If this waste is not removed regularly, the system will become sluggish, full of toxins, and vulnerable to serious health problems.

2. *Eat only when you are hungry.* Don't wait until you are famished, and don't eat just because there is food in front of you that looks or smells appealing. Listen to your body.

3. *Eat a balanced diet* of the five food groups discussed in this chapter and drink at least four glasses of water a day.

4. *Avoid fad diets.* If you need to lose weight, consult a qualified nutritionist or your physician.

5. *Reduce consumption of all highly processed foods:* white, brown, or raw sugar; corn syrup and sugar syrups; white rice and flour; salts; chemical additives; and artificial preservatives.

6. *Avoid all fried foods,* and all commercially produced foods like popcorn, potato chips, etc.

7. *Avoid all stimulants and depressants,* including alcohol, coffee, tobacco, chocolate, cocoa and hot pepper. They offer little or nothing nutritionally and can inhibit and even damage the autonomic nervous system.

8. *Beware of so-called natural cereals.* Although there are some good ones to be found in health-food stores, most of them contain brown sugar (no better than white sugar), salt, and other highly refined ingredients. And in many cases, synthetic preservatives have been added to the materials in which the cereals are packaged.

9. *Do not eat when in pain or when emotionally upset.* When you put food into a body that is not calm and ready for digestion, you are inviting indigestion, headaches, and other imbalances.

10. *Don't eat when you are in a hurry.* Eat slowly and chew your food well. The teeth and the mouth are the first organs of digestion. When food is chewed well, the stomach's digestive function is made easier. Also, people who eat slowly are likely to eat less. They get more nutritional benefit from the food they eat and are less likely to gain weight.

11. *Don't eat when you are exhausted* or immediately after hard work. Give the body an opportunity to build up the energy necessary to do the job of digestion efficiently.

12. *Do not drink liquids that are extremely hot or cold.* This can produce irritation in the digestive tract as well as muscle cramps.

13. *Read food labels carefully.* Most frozen vegetables contain salt or sauces or both. That a label reads "natural" or "no chemicals or preservatives added" does not necessarily indicate high quality. Many undesirable ingredients, such as white sugar and white flour, can be included that are not considered chemicals or preservatives. So-called dietetic foods containing artificial sweeteners such as saccharine and sorbital should also be avoided.

14. *Do not overcook vegetables and fruits.* This robs them of their nutrients. A steamer is an excellent investment.

15. *Add more raw fruits and juices to your diet.* A juice extractor, a blender, or a food processor, can provide rich and exotic liquid nourishment from fresh fruits and vegetables. Before blending different juices, check with a knowledgeable nutritional consultant as some foods are not compatible with one another.

Remember: *Moderation and balance are the key to healthy living. Too much of anything can be harmful. Find out what your body needs, learn the nutritional value and function of different foods, and then give your body what it needs for vital functioning.*

CHAPTER 11

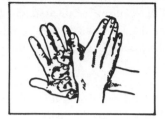

STAYING BEAUTIFUL THROUGH FACIAL MASSAGE

Some people are blessed with a well-designed face and body that are accidents—a lucky combination of genes. But deep and enduring beauty emanates from within and is the reflection of a peaceful mind and a healthy body. With care and effort, this true beauty is available to all of us. Self-analysis is the first step. How are your mental attitudes affecting your appearance? What about your diet? Are you getting enough exercise? Are you getting enough rest? Do you take proper care of your skin and hair? Do you have any personal habits that are damaging your appearance?

What you think and how you feel make a strong imprint on your face and body. Generally, your face is the clearest indication of your state of mind. Negative emotions such as persistent jealousy, anger, fear, and depression inhibit or tax vital bodily functions and put a stress on the entire system. This stress brings about a pinched and strained look in the face, unattractive lines, dulled eyes, and a variety of skin problems.

Positive feelings such as love and compassion—for yourself as well as others—tend to invigorate your body, increase the flow of blood, and bring a radiant glow to your expression. Smiles, which are nature's way of helping us communicate pleasure and happiness, not only make us look more attractive but also increase the circulation of blood in the face and improve muscle tone. This improves skin texture, prevents wrinkles, and keeps the facial contours from sagging. A smile is a truly wondrous thing.

Your body, especially your weight and your posture, reveals how you feel about yourself. Have you been promising yourself to lose ten pounds but just haven't been able to stick with a diet? The next time you walk past a window or mirror, take a good look at yourself. Do you like what you see? Do you look confident and relaxed, or anxious and uptight? Is your body balanced and your head erect, or do you hunch your shoulders, extend your pelvis, tilt your body to one side, hang your head? These and other distortions make you less attractive.

Massage, as well as the other activities in this book—water balancing, exercise, proper nutrition and tension reducing practices—when used regularly, will make you more attractive by making you healthier, stronger, and more relaxed. Visualization and other relaxation techniques (see Chapter 12, page 215) will help calm your emotions and allow inner peace and harmony.

Sound eating habits provide the basic elements for a healthy body and are a prerequisite for good skin and strong muscles, bones, teeth, hair, and nails. One of the greatest enemies of a beautiful appearance is overprocessed food and junk food. No cosmetics can improve your looks if your diet is filled with preservatives, sugar, and synthetic food colorings and flavorings.

Regular exercise strengthens and tones muscles and contributes to good posture. It will also improve circulation, distribute nutrients throughout the body, and regulate the elimination of waste, all of which help to clear your complexion and brighten your eyes. Exercise controls weight by burning up calories and reducing your appetite and brings about a general sense of physical and mental well-being.

The water-balancing techniques described in Chapter 9 can help improve circulation, cleanse and purify the skin, and stimulate or sedate the nervous system. When added to a sound nutrition and exercise regimen, they provide a final touch that completes the glow of health.

Though our massage techniques have proved to be wonderfully effective in enhancing personal appearance, in the absence of good nutrition and exercise, they will have only a limited beautifying effect. But as part of a total program of self-care, our techniques will make you look as good as they make you feel.

Facial Massage

Two basic beauty requirements are good circulation, which brings good coloring and good skin tone, and strong muscles, which keep the face and neck from sagging. The following ten-step facial massage will help to increase circulation, relax tense muscles, and tone flaccid muscles throughout the face and neck. You may either do the entire massage at one time or do it a bit at a time throughout the day, which ever fits your temperament and schedule. It takes about ten minutes.

With the exception of step 6, the massage involves firm Vital Force Contacts applied to different parts of the face. Place your elbow (or elbows, in some steps) squarely on a table in a comfortable position. Rest the specific part of your face on your finger (or fingers) and gently lean your face into your hand, while holding your arm stiff. Do not apply force with your hand. Hold the pressure for about fifteen seconds, release, and then repeat two more times.

Points for Facial Massage

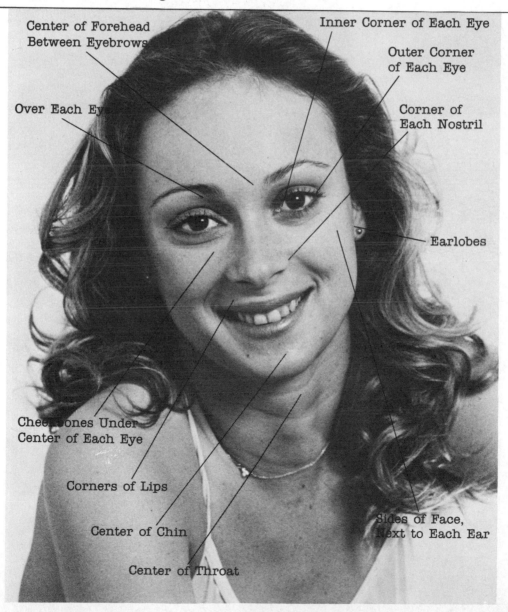

Step 1   Over the entire eye

Relieves tired eyes and relieves headaches.

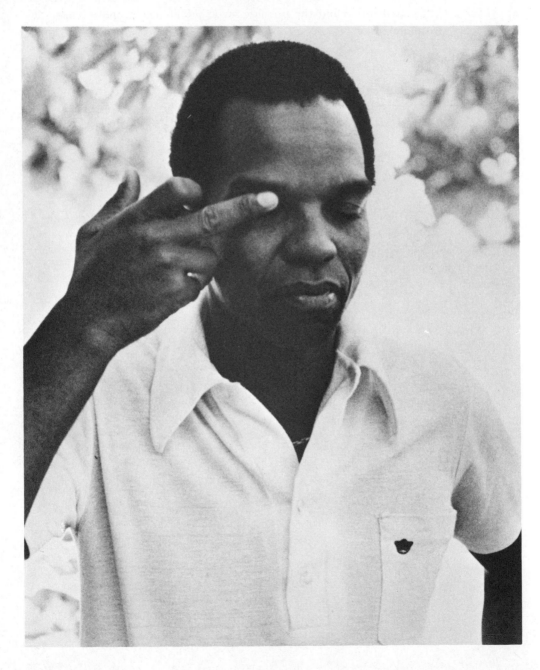

Step 2 Center of the forehead, between the eyebrows
Stimulates cell growth in face and aids in relieving headaches.

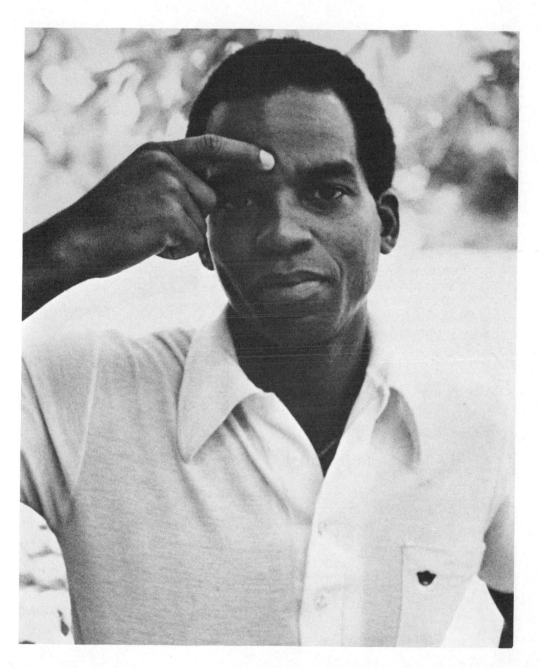

MASSAGEWORKS

Step 3   Inner and outer corners of the eyes

Relieves tension in eyes.

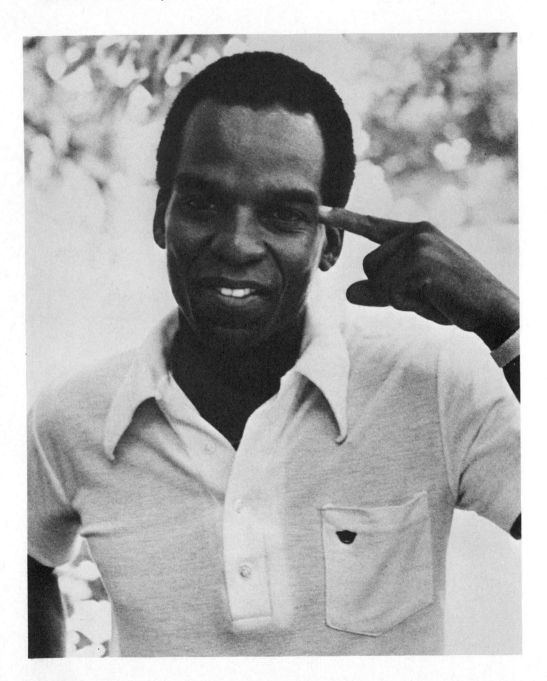

Step 4   Corners of the nostrils

Revitalizes the face by opening the nasal passages and allowing fresh oxygen into the body.

Step 5   Cheekbone, directly under centers of the eyes

Removes lines between the nose and mouth and stimulates circulation in lower part of face.

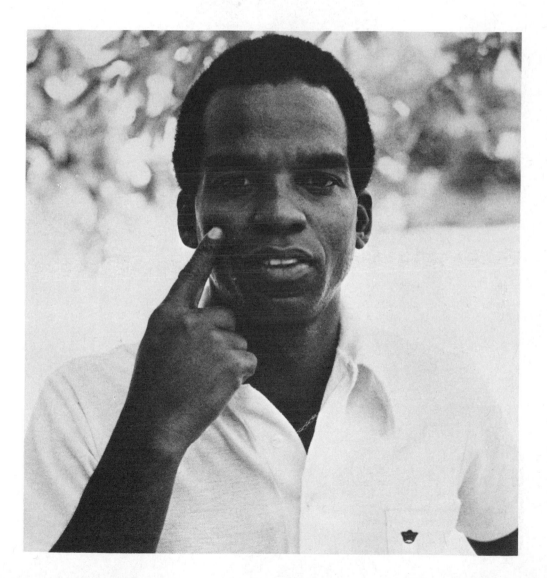

Step 6   Earlobe

Gently stroke the earlobes to remove dead skin from the face and beautify the ears, which in many ancient cultures were considered a source of beauty and wisdom.

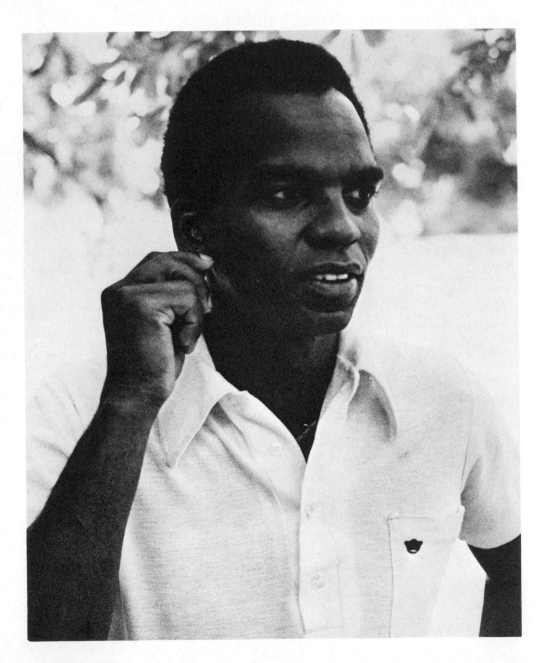

Step 7   Sides of the face, next to the ears

Brings luster to the skin and stops earaches and ringing in the ears.

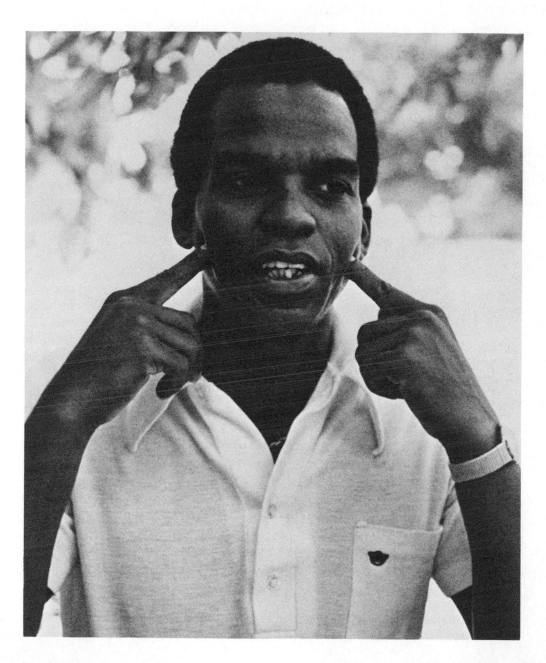

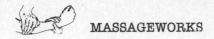

Step 8   Corners of the lips

Increases circulation in lips, making them moist and rosy.

Step 9   Center of the chin

Helps get rid of flabbiness in the neck under the chin, helps remove facial lines, and generally revitalizes the face.

Step 10   Center of the throat

Stimulates skin in neck area and clears and soothes the throat.

Exercises for the Face and Skin

Exercise of all kinds beautifies the skin by stimulating circulation, toning the muscles, and causing perspiration, which helps to eliminate waste materials from the body. The following are some specific exercises for the face and skin.

1. By reversing the flow of blood and the pull of gravity, head and shoulder stands are extremely beneficial for maintaining vibrant skin and a healthy head of hair. (See Chapter 8, page 167).

2. The lion pose is great for toning neck and facial muscles. Sit resting on your heels. Place your hands on your knees, palms up. Let the tension flow from your hands. Inhale deeply. Upon exhaling, open your mouth wide and stick out your tongue as though you were trying to reach your chin. Now tense your hands, your eyes, and the rest of your body. Hold this position for the count of seven; then release the entire body. Repeat this exercise seven times. (See page 124.)

3. To help prevent or eliminate lines around the mouth and in the lower part of the face, pucker your lips as if giving someone a big kiss. Hold this position for the count of seven and then let go. Repeat seven times.

4. This exercise will help firm up the jawline. Open your mouth wide, as if yawning. Close slowly. Now stretch the mouth, lips, and tongue to the right and then to the left. Repeat seven times.

5. Here's a good exercise to strengthen the muscles around the eyes. Look straight up to the ceiling as high as you can. Next bring your eyes back to the center and without moving your head look as far left as possible as though you are trying to look at your left

ear. Now look straight down at the tip of your nose. Look toward your right ear. Hold each for a count of ten.

6. Smile often. You can carry your smile with you all the time, wherever you go. Take advantage of every opportunity to laugh and smile with your family, your friends, and people you meet. And when you're alone, think of something funny, a pleasant memory, or a delightful fantasy. Then generate a smile that travels throughout your entire body. If you pay careful attention, you can actually feel its vibrations.

Skin Care

The skin, which is the body's largest organ, is both very tough and very delicate. Besides providing protection for the muscles, bones, and internal organs, it is one of the main vehicles for removing waste from the body. If the skin is not functioning properly, or is not properly cleansed, this waste material may clog the pores and cause skin problems. Skin eruptions of any kind are generally a sign that some form of pollution is affecting the system. When the eliminatory activity is improved and the clogged pores are reopened, the skin begins to breathe and function normally and the unwholesome condition begins to disappear.

To keep the system clean, drink plenty of water and fresh fruit juices, exercise regularly, have upper colonic irrigations periodically, and keep the surface of the skin clean and free of potentially damaging toxins. A loofah or some other natural fiber sponge or bath mitt is very good for removing dead skin and waste, stimulating cell growth, and uncovering the skin's natural luster.

Some skin disorders are due to emotional stress, which can interfere with various systems of the body. These problems can be cured only by unearthing and dealing with the basic cause.

Nutrients for Beauty

Diet is very important for maintaining a healthy, glowing skin. Substances such as alcohol, tobacco, caffeine, sugar, excessive salt, and artificial colorings, preservatives, and flavorings are ultimately destructive. Plenty of water, fruits, vegetables, unsalted nuts, grains, and fresh juices lead to a clear complexion. Vitamins A, E, and the B complex are particularly important (see Chapter 10).

Vitamin A	Builds blood, tissues, and membranes. Lubricates the skin. Prevents dandruff. Aids the growth of hair, nails, bones, and teeth. Protects against air pollution and helps rid the face of acne.
Vitamin B	(Thiamine) Guards against stress, fatigue, and depression.
Vitamin B_2	Aids eyesight.
Vitamin B_3	(Niacin) Softens the skin.
Vitamin B_5	(Pantothenic acid) Heals and soothes the skin. Prevents wrinkles. Thickens the hair.
Vitamin B_6	Strengthens the blood. Keeps hair from graying.
Vitamin B_9	(Folic acid) Is essential for formation of red blood cells.
Vitamin C	Helps fight skin infections.
Vitamin D	Helps bones, teeth, vision. Helps prevent acne.
Vitamin E	Is essential for circulation. Aids skin and hair.
Vitamin F	Aids in reproduction of cells.
Protein	Is essential for building and maintaining tissue.
Zinc	Can be helpful in relieving acne.
Iron	Builds blood.
Paba	Is helpful in various skin disorders. Protects the skin against cancer, sunburn, and eczema.
Sulfur	Is valuable for producing healthy hair, skin, and nails.

For a tasty and nutritious drink, try the following fresh vegetable juice mixes.

Juice # 1

6 parts carrot   (beta carotene in carrots is converted to vitamin A)

2 parts apple   (high in malic acid, which is good for the tissues)

1 part beet   (high in iron)

Juice # 2

6 parts carrot

2 parts spinach   (high in iron, vitamin E)

The Ultimate in Cosmetics

A youthful looking, graying Quaker lady was asked what she used to preserve her appearance. She replied calmly:

> I use for the lips, truth;
> for the voice, prayer;
> for the eyes, pity;
> for the hand, charity;
> for the figure, uprightness;
> for the heart, love.

CHAPTER 12

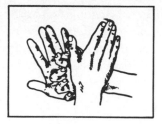

EASING YOUR MIND

To say that there is a direct relationship between the body and the mind is a serious understatement. When there is an imbalance in the mind, there is usually a corresponding one in the body.

A limited amount of stress and tension is a normal condition and is actually necessary for a balanced and productive life. But when the stress occurs in larger quantities than the body can handle, a pathological tension appears. It is this extreme tension that causes or contributes to health problems such as headaches, high blood pressure, heart conditions, certain arthritic conditions, skin problems, aches and pains throughout the body, and, in the opinion of some medical authorities, may even be a contributing factor to cancer.

While it would be totally impossible and really undesirable to eliminate all stress and tension from our lives, there are things we can do to minimize it and its effects.

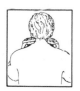

Take a Break

When you find yourself in a stress-producing situation, take a change of pace. If you are in a crowded hall filled with people, noise, and smoke, find a quiet, secluded place where you can be alone for a few moments. If you've been working alone for an extended period, call a friend for a chat or team up with a co-worker to discuss an idea or help resolve a problem.

Mini-breaks throughout the day can be very revitalizing. Listening to your favorite record, lying with your feet above your head, taking a short walk, doing a few minutes of stretching exercises, having a fifteen minute nap (if you are one of the lucky people who can do this)—any of these can help reduce tension and restore balance. The key is to find what works for you.

Do Deep Breathing and Relaxation Exercises

Usually, when we begin to get tense, our breathing becomes very shallow, interfering with circulation and reducing the amount of oxygen to the brain. This lack of oxygen can produce numerous symptoms—headache, irritability, inability to think or concentrate, and excessive fatigue. To relieve or prevent these symptoms, take a few seconds to do the following breathing exercise. Sit in a straight-back chair with both feet flat on the floor and the back of your open hands resting on your knees. (If you can't conveniently sit down, you can do the exercise while standing.) Close your eyes and inhale deeply through your nose to the count of four. As you inhale, first push out your stomach and then your chest gently. Hold your breath to the count of six. Then exhale to the count of eight, releasing the air first from your stomach and then from your chest. Do this three times. You'll probably be amazed at how light and relaxed it will make you feel, as well as energized.

Another simple relaxation exercise is to close your eyes while in a sitting position and let your head drop slowly toward your chest. Remain that way for a few moments then slowly straighten your head and open your eyes. Now close your eyes again and concentrate on relaxing various parts of your face.

When you are doing any relaxation exercise, remember to breathe deeply, slowly, and rhythmically.

A more profound relaxation exercise includes visualization, a technique that has long been recognized for its aid in relieving tired muscles and inducing feelings of relaxation, self-awareness, and confidence. Visualization for relaxation includes the following steps:

1. Find a quiet place where you can relax.

2. Sit in a comfortable, straight-back chair in the posture used for the breathing exercise or lie on your back with your legs lying straight and your arms relaxed at your sides.

3. Close your eyes and breathe deeply three times, using the 4-6-8 count. With each exhalation, visualize the tension leaving your entire body.

4. While breathing deeply, slowly, and rhythmically, picture the part of your body where you are holding an excessive amount of tension, such as your shoulders, lower back, arms—wherever you feel uncomfortable or in pain.

5. With each exhalation, visualize the tension leaving that area. With each inhalation, see the area becoming soothed and relaxed by the energy that is flowing into it.

6. Continue until you feel relief in that area and feel relaxed and energized.

7. Now take a deep breath and then slowly exhale, gradually opening your eyes as you do. Before moving, sit quietly for a few seconds.

Visualize a Pleasant Scene

Another form of visualization involves recreating mental pictures of scenes that you have found relaxing or peaceful or that have brought you happiness. White-capped ocean waves, a field of wild flowers, a walk on a country road, an evening with friends, a happy moment with a loved one—remembering these and other scenes can bring a glow to your expression, serenity to your thoughts, and relaxation to your body.

Visualization can be done just about any time and any place. All you need to do is close your eyes, get in a relaxed position, then visualize something that brings you pleasure. Some people find that it helps to put them to sleep at night. Others find it a great way to help start the day before getting out of bed. We have found it to be a particularly effective way for ending a bodywork session.

Meditation

Meditation can be defined in many ways. However, there is little disagreement about the fact that it is one of the most powerful means of taking control of the mind and body and enabling an individual to function at the highest level. Meditation is a process of focusing visual imagery wherever it is needed so that stress, tension, and emotional imbalances can be clarified and eliminated.

Learning Visualized Meditation

Find a quiet room and/or area where you may remain from five to twenty-five minutes

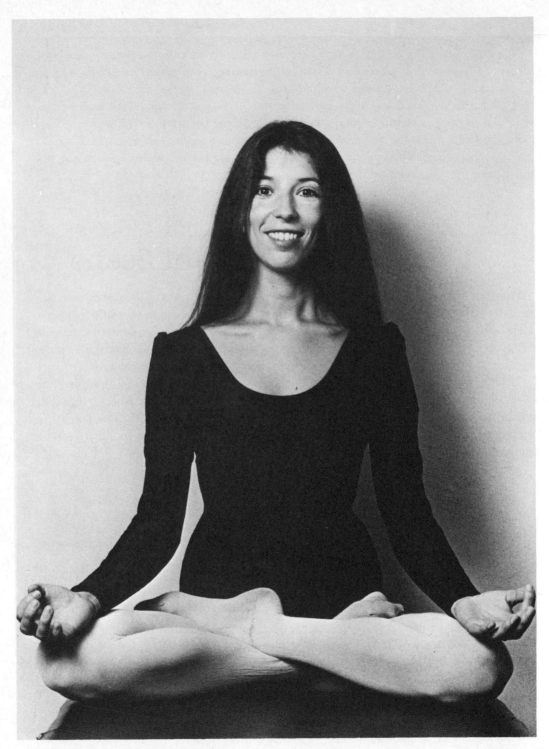

Learning visualized meditation

without being disturbed. If sitting on a chair or in a cross-legged position on the floor, place your hands on your thighs. If lying down, your arms should be placed on your side. Closing your eyes slowly, create a deep and relaxed breathing pattern, actually feeling the breath coming into your lower abdomen. As your breathing becomes regular, direct your attention to this full relaxing breath. Now create a visual image in your mind of a garden, waterfall, or beach—something very pleasant with color and sound. As you place this image fully into focus, your imagery combined with the subtlety and depth of the vital force balancing of the breath will bring about a greater self awareness and feeling of health and well-being. If your mind begins to wander from the image you have created simply return to that beach or waterfall as soon as you become aware of the diversion. You may expand the meditation environment by playing many of the wonderful and soothing tapes available which simulate the sound of the roaring tide, the waterfall or the droplets of falling rain. When you begin to come out of your visualized meditation keep your eyes closed while becoming aware of your surroundings. Slowly move your hands and feet and begin to wiggle the fingers and toes. After stretching your arms and legs and all of your muscles you may open your eyes.

Music

Sound is pervasive. It's with us in some form or another from the moment we awaken until we go to sleep. The vibrational patterns caused by sound have a direct effect on our body and can cause us to be irritable, uncomfortable, relaxed, or energized.

Sound, particularly music, has a profound influence on us and, in addition to influencing our emotions, can affect metabolism, alter breathing patterns, affect blood pressure, influence brain activity, influence internal secretions, and cause chemical changes in the body.

In general, music that is rhythmic, such as disco, reggae, popular dance music, or marches, is stimulating to the body and has an uplifting effect, and is good to exercise by. Many people who are slow starters in the morning find it very helpful to listen to dance music while they are taking a brisk shower to help get the blood circulating and the adrenalin flowing. It can also help lift you out of a blue or depressed mood.

Music that is slow and calm, with a predominance of mellow strings and soft piano, can relax, sooth, ease pain and tension, and aid digestion.

To relieve a headache, put on your favorite piece of soothing music, lay back, close your eyes, and put a cool pack on your forehead. Then just give yourself over to the music totally and let it fill your mind and your body.

The effects of music can vary from person to person since people have different reactions based on their genetic, cultural, and social influences. With a little experimentation, you'll be able to find music that is therapeutic for you as well as enjoyable. When selecting music to accompany bodywork, always choose music that is unobtrusive and relaxing to the person receiving the massage.

Biofeedback

Biofeedback is based on the principle that we can become aware of bodily functions that are usually considered unconscious and that through this awareness we can learn to control them. By becoming aware of breathing, heart rate, blood pressure, or muscle tension, we can consciously direct these functions in a way that improves our total health.

Biofeedback is done by machines that measure our brain's electrical signals. These machines feed back our biological processes. Although biofeedback instruments require an instructor or practitioner during the early learning stages, they can be used independently once the technique has been mastered.

Biofeedback can be used in conjunction with massage to help control headaches, lower backache, nervous tension, various muscle disorders, insomnia, and other conditions. It is probably best known as an adjunctive treatment for high blood pressure.

We are living in a stress-ridden society, and to totally eliminate stress from our lives is neither possible nor desirable. The key is to understand yourself and what creates stress for you. When stress occurs, how do you react? How is it manifested in your body? Do you get a headache, a backache, tension in your shoulders or chest? Do you get suddenly overcome with fatigue? Become sensitive to your body and its signals. If you pay careful attention, it will tell you most of what you need to know. You must then learn what works for you. Is it a long, luxurious bath? A quiet walk in the woods? A period of meditation? Some soothing music in a softly lit room?

We owe it to ourselves and to the people we love to be well. A program of sound nutrition, exercise, bodywork, and various relaxation techniques tailored to our individual needs, taste, and life style will help us to maintain physical and emotional fitness.

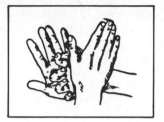

CHAPTER 13

BE AN INFORMED CONSUMER: WHERE TO GET A MASSAGE

Receiving a massage can be among the most relaxing experiences. Touch itself is extremely healing, and when applied skillfully by a sensitive person, it provides a unique feeling of well-being. Still, many people are confused about where they can obtain a massage or hands-on bodywork from skilled, well-trained practitioners. When you are interested in specialized bodywork such as polarity or shiatsu, it is good to know where to call or write for information about certified practitioners. The list below—not meant to be an endorsement of any particular technique—names centers and institutes that you may contact to learn more about various techniques and to receive referrals.

Once you have located a massage or bodywork therapist there are a number of ways that you may determine his or her qualifications.

1. When you call for information the therapist should answer your questions in a clear manner. They should know the specific benefits of the technique they are offering and be willing to certify their training. Many bodywork systems are controversial; however, the most important factor is that the therapist clearly understands the philosophy of the approach he or she is offering. Avoid any therapist who makes exaggerated claims or attempts to hard-sell you over the phone. Inquire about fees *before* you make the appointment.

2. When making appointments find out if the therapist makes home visits, and ask if a home visit costs more than an office visit.

3. Be sure that the therapist and his/her office is neat and clean. Offices should be free of distasteful odors.

4. The practitioner should show you the type of equipment he or she uses, the lighting used during the session, and the dressing room and shower facilities.

5. The best bodywork practitioners will wash their hands at the start of each massage and again at any time that the session is interrupted. The therapist should use clean linen for each client or change physiotherapy paper between clients.

6. A good practitioner will always be polite and patient and always will have a genuine interest in your well-being.

Massage has received a bad reputation because of untrained practitioners who give "sexual bodyrubs" and the like. The fact is that massage and bodywork techniques are applied in thousands of offices and hospitals by well-trained and licensed professionals. It would take a hundred books to describe all the case histories of people who, after years of stress, tension, back problems, headaches, and major medical disorders, finally found relief after receiving massage and bodywork from one of the highly skilled, well-trained and caring practitioners.

ALEXANDER TECHNIQUE

The American Center for the Alexander
  Technique, Inc.
142 West End Ave.
New York, NY 10023
(212) 799-0468

931 Elizabeth St.
San Francisco, CA 94114
(415) 282-8967

AMMA

Wholistic Center of Manhasset
50 Maple Place
Manhasset, NY 10030
(516) 627-0309

APPLIED KINESIOLOGY

International College of Applied Kinesiology
542 Michigan Building
Detroit, MI 48226
(313) 962-6484
George Goodheart, D.C., Founder

BIOFEEDBACK

Biofeedback Instrument Co.
255 W. 98th St.
New York, NY 10025
Mr. Philip Brotman, Pres.

Biofeedback Society of America
Psychiatry C 268
University of Colorado Medical Center

4200 E. 9th Ave.
Denver, CO 80220
(303) 394-7054
Francine Butler, Executive Director

Lawrence/Harrison Institute
Suite 1206
1990 Broadway
New York, NY 10023

Southern California Society for Psychical
  Research
170 South Beverly Drive
Beverly Hills, CA 90212
(213) 276-4523

CHIROPRACTIC

American Chiropractic Association
2200 Grand Ave.
Des Moines, IA 50312
(515) 243-1121

International Chiropractora Assoc.
741 Brady Street
Davenport, IA 52808
(319) 322-4447
B. Nordstrom, D.C., Public Information
Director

CHUA K'A

Arica New York
235 Park Ave.
New York, NY 10003
(212) 460-5455

MUSCULAR THERAPY
(THE BENJAMIN SYSTEM)

Muscular Therapy Institute Inc.
910 West End Ave.
New York, NY 10025

Sacro Occipital Research Society International
  (SORSI)
P.O. Box 338
Nebraska City, NE 68410

NAPRAPATHY

National College of Naprapathy
3330 N. Milwaukee Ave.
Chicago, IL 60641
(312) 282-5717

OSTEOPATHY

American Academy of Osteopathy
2630 Airport Road
Colorado Springs, CO 80910
(303) 632-7164
Louis W. Astell, Executive Director

American Osteopathic Association
212 East Ohio St.
Chicago, IL 60611
(312) 944-2713

North American Academy of Manipulative
  Therapy
c/o C. R. Hooper, M.D., D.O.
12238 113th Ave., Suite 106
Youngstown, AZ 85363
(602) 933-8787

MASSAGEWORKS

POLARITY THERAPY

Lawrence/Harrison Institute
Box 1206
1990 Broadway
New York, NY 10023
(212) 307-1399

Pierre Pannetier Polarity Center
401 North Glassell St.
Orange, CA 92666
(714) 532-3035
Pierre Pannetier, Director

Polarity Wellness Center
10 Leonard St.
New York, NY 10013
(212) 226-1087

SHIATSU

Shiatsu Education Center of America
52 W. 55th St.
New York, NY 10019
(212) 582-3424

SWEDISH MASSAGE

The American Massage and Therapy
 Association
P.O. Box 1270
Kingsport, TN 37662
(615) 245-8071

Boulder School of Massage Therapy
2855 Walnut
Boulder, CO 80302

Massage Guild of California
3119 Clement St.
San Francisco, CA 94121
(415) 668-0550

New York Society of Medical Masseurs
Box 1024
New York, NY 10019

ROLFING

The New York Center for Structural
 Integration and Structural Patterning
165 West 91st St. #8E
New York, NY 10024
(212) 724-6677

New York School of Rolfing
P.O. Box 758
Old Chelsea Station
New York, NY 10011
(212) 620-0931

Rolf Institute
P.O. Box 1868
Boulder, CO 80302
(301) 449-5903
Richard A. Stenstadvold, Executive Director

THERAPEUTIC TOUCH

American Holistic Nursing Association
Box 116
Telluride, CO 81435
(303) 728-4575

Center for Continuing Education in Nursing
New York University
Division of Nursing
429 Shimkin Hall
Washington Square
New York, NY 10003
(212) 598-3921

East/West Academy of the Healing Arts
P.O. Box 31211
San Francisco, CA 94131
(415) 285-8400

TOUCH FOR HEALTH

Touch for Health Foundation
1174 N. Lake Ave.
P.O. Box 751
Pasadena, CA 91104
(213) 794-1181

TRAGER

Inner Arts Center for Personal Growth
42 Pleasant St. #1
Northhampton, MA 01060

ZONE THERAPY AND REFLEXOLOGY

California Institute of Reflexology
275 Summitt Ave.
Mill Valley, CA 94941
(415) 383-4520

National Reflexology Association
414 25th St.
Virginia Beach, VA 23451
(804) 422-9090

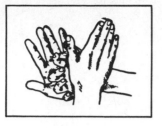

GLOSSARY

abduction   movement of a part of the body away from the midline

abrasion   a superficial skin wound as a result of scraping skin against a hard or rough surface

acute   of sudden or abrupt onset

adduction   movement of a limb toward the body midline

adhesion   fibrous bands of tissue that help body parts adhere to each other

aerobic   stimulating to the respiratory and circulatory systems

agonist muscle   a muscle in state of contraction

amino acid   a protein which performs a specific role in a particular biochemical process in the body

antagonist muscle   a muscle working in opposition to another muscle

anterior   located toward the front of the body

arteriosclerosis   hardening of the walls of the arteries

atrophy   an emaciation or wasting of tissues, organs or body parts

autonomic nervous system   the part of the nervous system that regulates bodily functions, such as temperature, respiration and glandular activity

biochemical   having to do with the chemistry of the substances involved in the life processes of any living organism

blockage	a limitation of freedom
body armor	patterns in the musculoskeletal system which are reflections of emotional patterns
bunion	a swelling of the bursa of the big toe
bursa	a small connective tissue-lined sac filled with synovial fluid, found at the joints and acting as cushions
bursitis	an inflammation of the bursae
calcaneus	bone of the heel
callus	development of thick skin where there is excess friction or pressure
cartilage	hard, connective tissue found at the ends of bones which absorbs shock and prevents direct wearing of the bones
charley horse	a contusion of the quadricep muscle group characterized by muscle cramping and pain
chronic	long-standing or recurring
collagen	a type of connective tissue
congenital	existing at birth but not hereditary
contraindicated	not advisable, as use may cause problems
contusion	a bruising of body tissue without a break in the skin
counterirritant	a substance applied to the skin which produces an analgesic effect
cramp	a painful contraction or spasm of a muscle
diaphragm	a broad sheet of muscle with attachments at the lower ribs, lumbar vertebrae and sternum, having its action influenced by breathing
disc	a pad of cartilage located between each vertebrae
dislocation	the movement of a bone from its normal position
energy fields	vibrational or electromagnetic pathways
equilibrium	a state of balance or harmony
esoteric	intended for or understood by a small group of people, often applied in mysticism
eversion	turning outward, away from the body midline

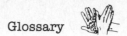

fascia	fibrous tissue that encloses, supports and separates muscles
flaccid	lacking firmness or tone
flexion	a bending movement which is directly opposed to the normal extension
fracture	a broken bone
hammer toe	a condition in which the big toe points upward and the second and third toes point downward
hemorrhage	bleeding
hernia	the protrusion of an organ or part of an organ through the tissue which normally surrounds and contains it
housemaid's knee	swelling of the prepatellar bursa, causing pain
hyperextension	overextension, excessive extension of a body part
hypertension	excessive stress and the buildup of tension, causing high blood pressure, headaches, etc.
inflammation	the reaction of tissues to injury or disease, characterized by redness, pain and swelling
inversion	a turning inward, toward the body midline
isometric	a way of contracting the muscles while maintaining the length of the muscles
kinesiology	the study of body motion and its relationship to the brain, nerves and muscles
lactic acid	a substance formed in the breakdown of glycogen in the muscles and found in fatigued muscles
lateral	outer side, away from the body midline
law of similars	the concept that certain parts and organs of the body are related to other parts by virtue of their similar shape (e.g. the sacrum and the calcaneus, the buttocks and the calf muscles)
ligament	band of fibrous tissue connecting and giving stability to bones at the joints
malleolus	a protruding bone found at the ankle joint
massage	rubbing of the body for therapeutic purpose
medial	inner side, toward the body midline

MASSAGEWORKS

membrane	a thin, pliable layer of tissue covering or separating body structures and organs
meniscus	a crescent-shaped cartilage located in the knee joint
metabolism	all physical, chemical and energy changes that take place within the body
multiple sclerosis	a degenerative disease of the central nervous system
muscle fatigue	a state in which a muscle has lost its power to contract
neurological	pertaining to the nervous system
orthopedist	a physician treating disorders of the skeletal system
osteopath	a physician using therapeutic bone manipulation in addition to other medical procedures
osteoporosis	a condition characterized by the loss of calcium from and porosity of the bones, common to the elderly
phlebitis	inflammation of a vein, usually caused by blockage of the vein
physiotherapy	the treatment of disease through the use of water, air, heat, massage, exercise or other physical forms of therapy
plantar	having to do with the sole of the foot
poliomyelitis	an infectious disease, causing paralysis of the muscles
psychogenic stress	stress which is triggered by the autonomic nervous system and is psychologically-oriented
pulse	throbbing or beat caused by expansion and contraction of the arterial walls
quadriceps	the muscle group located in the front of the thigh
range of motion	the fullest normal amount of extension and flexion of a body part at its joint
referred pain	pain felt in a part of the body other than the part which is actually the source of the pain
reflex	an involuntary response to a stimulus, a pressure point which affects another area in the body
resistance	the force opposing the natural flow
rolling	a condition in which the inner border of the foot falls inward

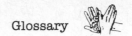

rotation	the turning of a bone at its axis
scoliosis	an abnormal lateral curvature of the spine
shin splints	a straining of the muscles of the lower leg, causing pain
spasm	an involuntary and sudden muscular contraction
sprain	the tearing of supporting ligaments
spur	a bony projection
strain	the pulling or tearing of muscle fibers
symptomatic	referring to the indication, sensation or appearance of a disorder or disease
synergy	coordination of muscles or organs by the nervous system so that a specific action can be performed
temporomandibular joint	the joint at the junction of the temporal bone and the mandible (jaw), commonly called the TMJ
tendon	strong, fibrous tissue which connects muscle to bone
tendonitis	the inflammation of a tendon
therapeutic	having healing or curative powers
thrombosis	the formation or presence of a blood clot
ultrasound	mechanical vibrations which generate local heat to an area of the body for therapeutic use
uric acid crystallization	the deposit of uric acid, a waste product, in a part of the body
varicose veins	abnormal stretching and swelling of the walls of the veins usually occurring in the legs and caused by excessive standing, obesity or pregnancy
vital force	sum total of the body's energy or life force
vitality	life force or energy, healthy and essential
wholistic/holistic	a state in which, in nature, the individual (entity) or other complete organism cannot be reduced to the sum of its parts, but functions as a complete unit
yoga	the practice of exercise in various postures, emphasizing the harmony of body and mind

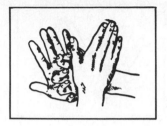

BIBLIOGRAPHY

There are hundreds of fine works on health care and massage; however, there are certain books that stand out as examples of clarity and vision. Below we have listed some of the works that we have found to properly fit this description.

Benjamin, Ben. *Sports Without Pain.* New York: Summit Books, 1979.

Conti, Gustave V. *Structural Analysis: Osteopathic Manipulative Management of Spine and Extremities.* Gustave V. Conti, nd.

Haehl, Richard. *Massage: Its History, Technique and Therapeutic Uses.* Reprint from the Hahnemannian Institute. Philadelphia: Dunlap Printing, 1898.

Kaslof, Leslie J., ed. *Wholistic Dimensions in Healing.* New York: Doubleday, 1978.

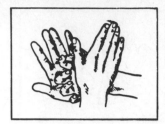

INDEX

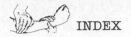 INDEX

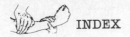 **INDEX**

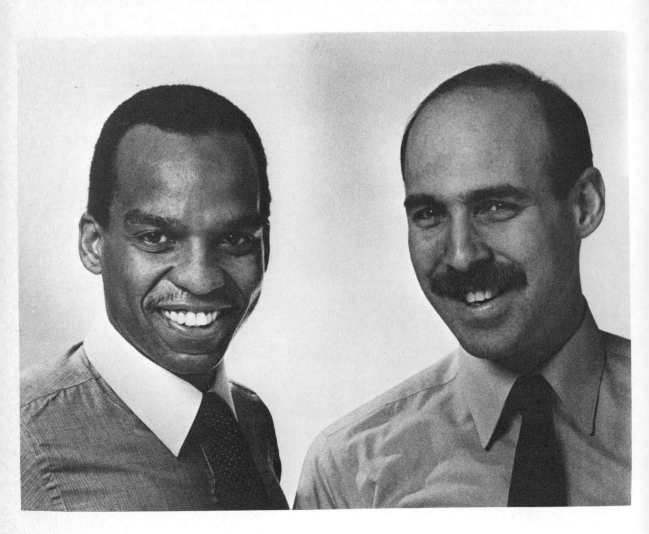

AUTHORS' BIOGRAPHIES

D. Baloti Lawrence and Lewis Harrison are pioneers in the field of holistic health. At the Lawrence/Harrison Institute in New York City, they serve clients ranging from professional athletes to corporate executives. Their innovative approach to health maintenance concentrates on preventing and relieving physical problems that can result from the types of work their clients do. Massage is used extensively in combination with visualization, sound and color therapy, and nutritional counseling.

The authors are both committed to health education. Baloti has taught at Morgan State College and Upsala College; lectured at Columbia University, the College of New Rochelle, Georgetown University, and the University of Iowa; and consulted for such organizations as the Veterans Administration and the U.S. Office of Education. Both Baloti and Lewis have made numerous appearances on radio and television to demonstrate massage and other health maintenance techniques. Baloti has also produced a film and audio-cassettes on self-help health techniques, while both have written articles on nutrition, herbology and massage for such publications as *Whole Life Times, Self*, the New York *Daily News, Essence*, and *The Massage Journal*. They are both licensed in several bodywork therapies.

For more information about the Lawrence/Harrison Institute, send a self-addressed, stamped envelope to 1990 Broadway, Box 1206, New York, NY 10023.